Dictionary of Evidence-based Medicine

©1998 Alain Li Wan Po

Radcliffe Medical Press Ltd
18 Marcham Road, Abingdon, Oxon OX14 1AA

British Library Cataloguing in Publication Data

A catalogue record for this book is available from the British Library.

ISBN 1 85775 305 4

Typeset by Advance Typesetting Ltd, Oxon
Printed and bound by Biddles Ltd, Guildford and King's Lynn

Preface

This book was conceived at one of the regular discussion meetings which we hold within the Centre for Evidence-Based Pharmacotherapy at the University of Nottingham. At the time, the group consisted of doctoral candidates in their first, second and third year of studies, mostly pharmacists by training, several hospital pharmacists and two post-doctoral fellows, one with a medical background (WYZ) and one with a statistical and biological sciences background (XYS). Each was working in the broad area of medicines assessment, pharmacoepidemiology and pharmacoeconomics (MAPP) research and all had as an objective the production of results which would be of value to practitioners of evidence-based medicine (EBM). Members therefore shared much of the same reading material. Yet with their multidisciplinary background, they had different levels of expertise in the subareas of our research focus.

At that meeting, several members of the group indicated that they would find helpful a glossary of terms commonly used in EBM. We agreed that they would produce a list of terms which they had some difficulty defining and in due course a list of some 50 terms appeared. It was interesting that the list included not only terms such as 'number needed to treat', 'meta-analysis' and 'effect size' which were essential for reading the EBM literature but also others such as 'multiattribute scale', 'allocative efficiency', 'construct', 'Markov modelling', 'hazard function' and 'Gompertz modelling'. Statisticians in our group found no problems with the statistical terminology but some pharmacists and doctors were ill prepared for it and vice versa when it came to pharmaceutical or clinical terminology. Dictionaries or glossaries available were too terse to provide the level of understanding being sought. As a result, I decided to write this dictionary which I expanded to become a notebook so that in addition to providing definitions, I could also provide some explanatory notes and references which I personally found useful when I first grappled with the relevant concepts. The reader is hence given the opportunity to read further.

Who, then, is this book aimed at? First, it is aimed at research students like my own and people like myself with a broad interest in the area of MAPP research and evidence-based medicine. However, I think that this book should have wider appeal. In particular, I feel that undergraduates and practitioners in a variety of health care disciplines (medicine, health economics, medical statistics, pharmacy, nursing and social sciences) will find it useful because health care literature is increasingly multidisciplinary and quick reference to the literature in cognate disciplines is often required. This extended dictionary is intended to serve as a convenient bridge.

It is impossible to do justice to the many who have contributed to the literature in this area. I have cited some but hope that those I have failed to acknowledge will understand. In particular, I hope that I have not distorted the meanings of the terms they first coined. If I have done so unjustifiably in certain cases, I would be pleased to have these, and any omissions, drawn to my attention so that they can be amended in any subsequent edition.

I wish to acknowledge members of my research group for sparking the idea for this book and for commenting on early drafts of the manuscript. I am particularly grateful to Darren Ashcroft, Christine Clark, Tim Kingscote-Davies, Nalinee Poolsup and Wei Ya Zhang for their comments which helped me to clarify many of my thoughts.

Alain Li Wan Po
Professor of Clinical Pharmaceutics
Centre for Evidence-Based Pharmacotherapy
University of Aston in Birmingham
August 1998

A

Ability to pay

Ability to pay is a criterion often used for determining the level of charges to try to make them fair. Most countries adopt this criterion for taxes by making them progressive in that those on higher income pay a higher proportion of their wages in taxes. In the UK, prescription charges are based on this criterion but with a cut-off point rather than use of a progressive scale (*see* **Benefits received** for comparison).

Absolute income hypothesis

The absolute income hypothesis states that the higher an individual's income, the lower his or her risk of mortality (Pritchett L, Summers LA (1996) Wealthier is healthier. *Journal of Human Resources.* **31**: 841–68).

Absolute risk (*see under* **Risk**)

Academic detailing

Academic detailing refers to university-based educational programmes designed to improve physicians' clinical decision making with a view to enhancing the quality and cost-effectiveness of health care. Such programmes, also known as **educational outreach** or **public interest detailing**, make use of behavioural science-based approaches adopted by pharmaceutical manufacturers to influence prescribing practices. Techniques used include (i) interviews to define baseline knowledge and motivations for current prescribing patterns; (ii) identification of target categories of physicians and their opinion leaders; (iii) defining clear educational and behavioural objectives; (iv) establishment of credibility through associations with well-respected organizations, citation of authoritative and unbiased sources of information and dispassionate presentation of opposing views while at the same time highlighting preferred options with justifications; (v) encouragement of active physician participation; (vi) use of concise and well-designed graphic educational material; (vii) highlighting and repeating of essential messages; (viii) provision of positive reinforcements in follow-up visits (Samurai SBA, Avon J (1990) Principles of educational outreach (academic detailing) to improve clinical decision making. *Journal of the American Medical Association*. **263**: 549–56).

ACBS (see Advisory Committee on Borderline Substances)

Activities of daily living
This term refers to measures of independence in the performance of five major personal care activities, specifically: bathing, dressing, eating, getting in and out of bed and using the toilet. Assessment of impairment of physical function is often undertaken using scales constructed from the five activities of daily living (Patrick DL, Erickson P (1993) *Health status and health policy*. Oxford University Press, Oxford).

Acquiescence response set
This term refers to the tendency of respondents to agree with statements of opinion regardless of content. For example, it is well known that in research aiming to gauge patient perception (e.g. patient satisfaction questionnaires), respondents to questionnaires sometimes respond positively to pairs of contradictory statements. Indeed, a small proportion of respondents are known to agree with all or nearly all items on questionnaires used in such studies. Such poor internal consistency therefore needs to be accounted for if the results of the studies are to be meaningful. Exclusion of acquiescent patients prior to analysis is not justifiable as a new source of bias may be introduced in the selection of such individuals. Moreover, restricting analysis to the subset of respondents from which acquiescent responders have been eliminated would reduce the external validity or generalizability of the results as acquiescent individuals are often from socioeconomic disadvantaged groups. The use of balance scales (i.e. scales which include items which express both favourable and unfavourable items) is recommended to minimize bias introduced by acquiescent response set.

Adaptive design
An adaptive design is a type of clinical trial design in which the probability that a patient receives a given treatment is, at least partly, determined by the results obtained with patients so far. An example of such a design is the

play the winner. In a trial using this design, the next patient is allocated to the same treatment as the last one if it was successful and to the other treatment otherwise (Sen S (1997) *Statistical issues in drug development.* John Wiley, Chicago).

Administrative analysis

In a clinical trial, monitors are normally appointed to ensure that progress is being made according to plans. Patient enrolment, event rates and/or safety profile of the drug are checked to ensure that they are broadly as expected. Such analyses, which do not involve any formal statistical analyses, are referred to as administrative analyses.

Adverse drug reaction (ADR)

For marketed medicinal products, an adverse reaction to a drug is a noxious and unintended response which can plausibly be attributed to the drug at doses normally used in man for the prophylaxis, diagnosis or therapy of disease or modification of physiological function. The definition is broadened to include any dose of the drug when dealing with pre-approval clinical experience since at that stage the normal dose of the drug has yet to be defined. An ADR is said to be unexpected if its nature or severity is not consistent with the applicable product information. If the ADR is life-threatening or leads to death then it is clearly serious. The term 'life-threatening' is itself used when the ADR leads to hospitalization or prolongation of hospital stay, results in persistent or significant disability or in a congenital anomaly or birth defect. Note that the descriptor 'serious' is not synonymous with 'severe'. The latter refers to intensity of the experience (e.g. severe headache) rather than to its prognostic significance (Edward IR *et al.* (1994) Harmonisation in pharmacovigilance. *Drug Safety.* **10**: 93–102 and *see* **Type A reaction**).

Adverse event

An adverse event is any untoward occurrence in any subject given a pharmaceutical product, irrespective of whether or not a causal relationship can be established. The term is used synonymously with 'adverse experience'. An adverse event is said to be serious if it is life-threatening or leads to death (Edward IR *et al.* (1994) Harmonisation in pharmacovigilance. *Drug Safety.* **10**: 93–102).

Advisory Committee on Borderline Substances

The Advisory Committee on Borderline Substances (ACBS) is a non-statutory body of experts representing medical, pharmaceutical and dietetic opinion, first set up in 1971 to advise UK health ministers whether particular unlicensed substances, preparations or items (foods, dietary supplements and toiletries) should be treated as drugs which are prescribable at the expense of the National Health Service (paragraph 43 of Schedule 2 to the NHS (General Medical Services) Regulations 1992). The chairman and members of the Committee are appointed by the UK Secretary of State for Health and three other members are appointed by the Secretaries of State for Wales, Scotland and Northern Ireland.

The Committee's terms of reference include ensuring that substances, preparations or items which have a therapeutic use in the treatment of disease in the community can be provided as economically as possible under the NHS. Products which the Committee recommends may be regarded as drugs are published in the *Drug Tariff* and in the *British National Formulary*. Although the list has no legal force, it is widely followed by both health authorities and prescribers in the community (GPs).

The ACBS also advises the ministers on which products should not be prescribed at NHS expense either because they have not demonstrated a therapeutic use in treating disease in the community or because they do not meet a need as economically as possible. Such products are added to a negative list or blacklist (Schedule 10 to the NHS (General Medical Services) Regulations 1992) and GPs are legally barred from prescribing them at NHS expense though not on private prescriptions. The blacklist is given at part XVIIIA of the *Drug Tariff*. This blacklist also includes recommendations made by other committees, notably the Advisory Committee on NHS Drugs, and agreed by ministers.

Age-specific rate (see **Specific rate**)

Allocative efficiency (see under **Efficiency**)

Allostasis

Allostasis is the ability to achieve stability of body systems through change. Allostasis is essential to survival and is provided through the co-ordinated responses of the autonomic nervous system, the hypothalamic-pituitary axis, the cardiovascular system, the metabolic system and the immune system (McEwen BS (1998) Protective and damaging effects of stress mediators. *New England Journal of Medicine.* **338**: 171–9. Sterlin P, Eyer G (1988) Allostasis. A new paradigm to explain arousal pathology. In: Fisher S, Reason G (eds) *Handbook of life stress, cognition and health.* John Wiley, New York, pp. 629–49).

Alludes terms

In statistical terminology, notably that associated with experimental design, alludes terms are those which cannot be estimated independently because there are fewer independent points in the design than there are terms in the statistical model used.

Alpha spending approach

The alpha spending approach is one of the approaches to sequential trials in which the type I error rate is controlled by proposing a time path for spending the type I error rate allowed in the trial. This approach avoids having to specify prospectively the exact times at which the analyses must be undertaken (Lan KEG, Demotes DL (1983) Discrete sequential boundaries for clinical trials. *Biometrics.* **70**: 659–63).

Analytic epidemiology

Analytic epidemiology deals with testing hypotheses about risk factors and the occurrence of specific diseases.

Approval phase

The approval phase in the development of a therapeutic drug refers to the interval between submission of a new drug application (NDA) and marketing approval given by the licensing authority (FDA in the USA).

Arithmetic series

An arithmetic series is a sequence of numbers characterized by a constant difference (d) between each consecutive term. Such an *n* term series can be written as $a, a + d, a + 2d, \ldots, a+(n-1)d$ where *a* is the first term. The sum S_n of such a series is given by:

$$S_n = \frac{n}{2}(2a + (n-1)d)$$

As treated analysis (see Intention to treat analysis)

ASTRO-PUs

Prescriptions written by general practitioners and dispensed by pharmacists in England are sent to the Prescription Pricing Authority for pricing so that reimbursements can be made to the pharmaceutical contractors. The data held provide information on the number of prescriptions dispensed, the drugs dispensed, the dosage forms and the number of units dispensed but not the diagnosis. Age groupings are made broadly on the basis of prescription exemptions. Those under 16 and pensioners are exempt from payment. In drug utilization studies, it is useful to make adjustments to account for covariates which may influence prescribing. The ASTRO-PUs was a weighting scheme developed to make such adjustments. Eighteen age–sex groupings and one temporary resident group were defined in that scheme which has since been further developed to facilitate comparisons at the therapeutic group level (see **STAR-PUs**) (Roberts S, Harris CM (1993) Age, sex and temporary resident originated prescribing units (ASTRO-PUs): new weightings for analysing prescribing of general practices in England. *BMJ*. **307**: 485–8).

Audit

An audit is an official examination, usually of accounts, to assess how well a business or service is functioning. Auditing is now usually thought of in terms of a cycle whereby practice is assessed by independent observers and checked against prospectively set standards. Any deficiency is highlighted and brought to the attention of the appropriate managers so that appropriate changes can be agreed upon and implemented. Subsequently, practice is again observed to complete the cycle (Figure 1). High standards of practice can therefore be achieved and maintained through this system of quality assurance.

Audit Commission

The UK Audit Commission was established in 1983 to appoint and regulate the external auditors of local authorities in England and Wales. In 1990, its responsibilities were extended to include the National Health Service, which provides health care for all UK citizens. Its auditors are required to examine arrangements made by health authorities for securing economy, efficiency and effectiveness in areas of expenditure for which they are responsible. One of the Commission's most recent reports on the

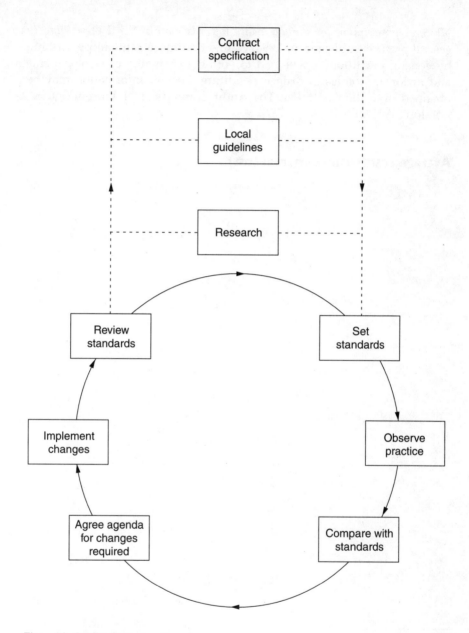

Figure 1 Audit: Clinical audit cycle

NHS, *A prescription for improvement. Towards more rational prescribing in general practice* published in 1994, claims that more rational prescribing by general practitioners will lead to both better quality care for patients and major economies in drug expenditure. Further information may be obtained from the Controller, The Audit Commission, 1 Vincent Square, London SW1P 2PN.

Average cost (see Incremental cost)

B

Balanced design

In an experiment, the effects of one or more predictor factors on one or more responses are followed. The factors can be set at different levels and various statistical designs can be used. A balanced experimental design is one in which low and high levels of any factor or interaction occur in equal numbers.

Bandolier

Bandolier is a monthly newsletter published by the Anglia and Oxford National Health Service (NHS) Executive in the UK. It focuses on evidence-based medicine, reviews relevant methodologies and reports on systematic reviews. It is distributed free within the UK NHS and may be accessed on the Internet (http://www.jr2.ox.ac.uk:80/Bandolier/).

Bayes, Thomas R

The Reverend Thomas Bayes (1702–61) was an English vicar at the Presbyterian Chapel in Tunbridge Wells, Kent. His fame is derived from his posthumously published paper, submitted on his behalf by a friend, Richard Price, describing how to update the probability of events in the light of new data (*see* **Bayes' theorem**). His work has led to the development of a whole new branch of statistics known as Bayesian statistics or Bayesian inference (Bayes T (1763) An essay towards solving a problem in the doctrine of chances. *Philosophical Transactions of the Royal Society.* **53**: 370–418).

Bayes' factor (*see under* Bayes' theorem)

Bayes' theorem

Bayes' theorem, named after the Reverend Thomas Bayes, describes the procedure for updating the probability of some event as new evidence becomes available.

$$P(A|B) = \frac{P(B|A)P(A)}{P(B)}$$

where $P(A|B)$ = conditional probability of event A given that event B has occurred and $P(B|A)$ the conditional probability of B given A.

In diagnostic testing the theorem can be expressed as:

$$P(D|+T) = \frac{P(D)P(+T|D)}{P(D)P(+T|D) + P(\bar{D})P(+T|\bar{D})}$$

where D = disease, $+T$ = positive test, $P(\bar{D})$ = probability of no disease and $P(D|+T)$ = probability of disease given that (or conditional on) the test is positive; $P(+T|D)$ = probability of positive test given the presence of the disease; $P(+T|\bar{D})$ = probability of positive test given that the disease is absent.

The theorem can be generalized to:

$$P(E_i|A) = \frac{P(A|E_i)P(E_i)}{\sum_{j=1}^{n} P(A|E_i)P(E_i)}$$

where $E_1, E_2, \ldots, E_n$ are mutually exclusive and exhaustive events and A is any other event in the same domain.

Bayes' theorem can also be expressed in terms of **odds**, as follows:

$$\frac{P(A|B)}{P(\bar{A}|B)} = \frac{P(B|A)}{P(B|\bar{A})} \times \frac{P(A)}{P(\bar{A})}$$

The equation states that the posterior odds ($\frac{P(A|B)}{P(\bar{A}|B)}$) in favour of A is the product of the Bayes' factor ($\frac{P(B|A)}{P(B|\bar{A})}$) and the prior odds ($\frac{P(A)}{P(\bar{A})}$) in favour of A. The Bayes' factor is hence the ratio of the likelihood of event A for observation B ($P(B|A)$) and the likelihood of event not A for observation B ($P(B|\bar{A})$). The **likelihood** of a model can be defined as the probability of the observations given that model (Figure 2).

Bayesian inference

Bayesian inference uses Bayes' theorem as a basis for making inference. Central to Bayesian inference is the concept of conditional probability. Unlike classic statistical inference, parameters are considered as random variables with their own statistical distributions rather than as fixed entities. In Bayesian statistical inference the observations are considered fixed while the parameters are not. In contrast, in classic statistical inference, the parameters are considered as fixed but the observations are not, although they are known.

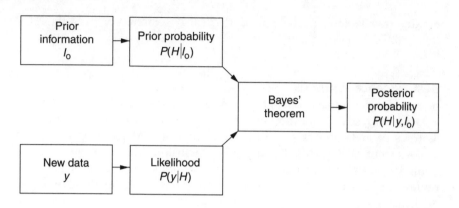

Figure 2 Bayes' theorem: Bayesian revision of probabilities given new data

Benefits received

Benefits received is a criterion used for assessing the fairness of various charges, particularly in relation to taxes. Property taxes are often set to meet this criterion since larger properties would utilize more of public services, such as garbage disposal and police protection (*see* **Ability to pay** for comparison).

Berkson's fallacy

Berkson's fallacy refers to the spurious correlation which may be observed between two diseases or between a disease and a risk factor arising from biased sampling (Berkson J (1946) Limitations of the application of four-fold table analysis to hospital data. *Biometrics Bulletin*. **2**: 47–53).

Best evidence

There is much controversy about what constitutes best evidence on which to base decisions in the health care context. There is wide agreement that for establishing efficacy, a well-designed and conducted randomized controlled trial (RCT) is the gold standard. However, it is also widely accepted that the results of RCTs may not generalize very well to the practice situation and other trial designs may be more appropriate (Green G, Wennberg J, Sackett D (1997) Best evidence. *BMJ*. **315**: 1636).

Best Evidence is also the name of an annually updated CD-ROM publication which includes articles from the American College of Physicians (ACP) Journal Club and editorials on various issues in clinical decision making (available from the British Medical Association or from the ACP (tel: +800-523-1546 ext. 2600).

Best evidence synthesis

Best evidence synthesis refers to the systematic review of the literature on a particular research question using an approach which combines the best features of **meta-analysis** and **narrative reviews.** At its heart is the use of consistent, well-justified and *a priori* inclusion criteria. Therefore, this approach is essentially the same as that adopted in a good **systematic review** and the terms can be used synonymously (Slavin RE (1995) Best evidence synthesis: an intelligent alternative to meta-analysis. *Journal of Clinical Epidemiology.* **48**: 9–18).

Beyren's-Fisher problem

The hypothesis testing for the equality of the means of two normal distributions known not to have the same variance is difficult using classic statistics. This problem is known as the Beyren's-Fisher problem. Of the various test statistics proposed, the one generally adopted is given by:

$$t = \frac{\bar{x}_1 - \bar{x}_2}{\sqrt{\frac{s_1^2}{n_1} + \frac{s_2^2}{n_2}}} \text{ and } df = \frac{(\frac{s_1^2}{n_1} + \frac{s_2^2}{n_2})^2}{\{\frac{(\frac{s_1^2}{n_1})^2}{(n_1 - 1)} + \frac{(\frac{s_2^2}{n_1})^2}{(n_2 - 1)}\}}$$

where $\bar{x}_1, \bar{x}_2, s_1^2, s_2^2, n_1, n_2$ are the means, variances and sizes of the samples of observations from the two populations. df is the degrees of freedom for the t distribution.

BGA

BGA is the abbreviation for Bundesgesundheitsamts, the Federal Health Office which acts as the German Drug Regulatory Agency.

Bias

Bias refers to the systematic deviation of an estimates from the true value. Unlike random variations round a true estimate, a biased estimate is one which is consistently lower or higher than the true value. For example, if a coin is fair and we flick it, say, 500 times and calculate the proportion of times it lands heads, we would expect this to be close to 0.5. If we repeat this experiment many times and ignore the occasions when the proportion is exactly 0.5, on average half of the time, the proportions will be on the low side of 0.5 and the other half on the high side. If the coin were loaded, then we would expect the two proportions to be unequal to an extent which will be proportional to the loading.

In clinical studies, two common sources of bias are (i) poor sampling leading to non-representative samples being assessed (e.g. estimating the efficacy of a smoking cessation aid in a general population using inpatient post-myocardial patients as a sampling frame) and (ii) flaw in the measurement method or process (e.g. use of a faulty sphygmomanometer in blood pressure measurement).

Information bias occurs when systematic differences are introduced in the measurement of the response. A well-known example is recall bias in case-control studies. Patients (cases) with, say, an adverse reaction are more likely to recall exposure to a suspected drug than are control subjects.

Non-response bias refers to bias which may be introduced when those who respond may differ systematically from non-responders. For this reason, those conducting surveys take great care to design their studies to minimize non-response and to make adjustments in their analyses to account for any non-response.

Protopathic bias (also referred to as reverse causality) is the term applied when a bias arises from misclassification, for example when general awareness of the study being carried out leads to exposure after the index date being reported more frequently in the case patients than in the controls.

Selection bias arises in comparative studies when the investigator inadvertently assigns patients with different characteristics which have a bearing on the outcome to the various groups. An often quoted example is that of a trial of a travel sickness remedy. Passengers were allocated to the control group and the ship's crew to the treatment group (the captain thought he could not afford to have travel-sick crew!).

Staging bias is a type of selection bias in which patients with different levels of disease severity are assigned in a biased way to the different treatment groups. This causes confounding by disease severity. In a review of comparative studies of radical prostatectomy and irradiation for the management of patients with early-stage prostate cancer, the authors found that patients who received radiation therapy tended to have more aggressive tumours than those who received surgery. Moreover, in the surgery group, surgery may be abandoned if examination of the regional lymph nodes early in the procedure reveals evidence of cancer spread. By expressing results in terms of survival for patients without spread at the time of surgery, surgical patients were bound to perform better than those subjected to radiation, a group which included patients with disseminated disease (Wasson J, Cushman C, Bruskewitz R *et al.* (1993) A structured literature review of treatment for localised prostate cancer. *Archives of Family Medicine.* **2**: 487–93).

Binary contingent valuation (*see under* Contingent valuation)

Binary variable
A variable for which there are only two outcomes (e.g. living status – dead or alive – or outcome of tossing a coin).

Binomial distribution
Consider a series of Bernoulli trials (i.e. each trial has only two outcomes). Suppose that the probability of success in each trial is the same and equal to p and that n trials are undertaken. If Y is the random variable representing the number of successes in the n trials, then Y follows the binomial probability distribution given by:

$$P(Y = y) = \binom{n}{y} p^y q^{n-y}$$

where y is an actual observation and $q = (1-p)$. An example which is easy to relate to is a series of tosses of the same coin. Each toss of the coin is a Bernoulli trial with probability of obtaining a head of 0.5 for a fair coin. y is the number of heads in the n trials.

$$\binom{n}{y} = \frac{n!}{y!(n-y)!}$$

Note that 0! is defined as 1. The binomial distribution has mean np and variance npq.

Binomial theorem
The binomial theorem gives the formula for expanding expressions of the form $(x + y)^n$:

$$(x+y)^n = \sum_{k=0}^{k} \binom{n}{k} x^k y^{n-k}$$

Bioavailability

Bioavailability is a term used to describe the absorption characteristics (rate and extent) of a drug from a formulation. The indices used for comparative purposes are the extent of absorption, usually assessed by area under the blood level–time curve (AUC), the maximum concentration achieved in the blood (C_{max}) and the time (T_{max}) taken to reach the C_{max}.

The term 'absolute bioavailability' is used when the bioavailability of a drug from a formulation is compared against that of a rapid intravenous equivalent dose. When the comparator is another dosage form administered by a route other than intravenous, the term 'relative bioavailability' is used.

For drugs not intended to be absorbed into the bloodstream, bioavailability may be assessed by measurements intended to reflect the rate and extent to which the active ingredient or active moiety becomes available at the site of action.

Bioequivalence studies

Bioequivalence studies are undertaken to compare the bioavailability of a drug from two formulations, usually with a view to showing that the two formulations are bioequivalent (i.e. have the same bioavailability). For systemic drugs, many drug regulatory authorities consider two formulations as being bioequivalent if the 90% confidence interval for the ratio of the area under the blood level–time curve (AUC) is in the range 0.80–1.25. Tighter ranges may be required for drugs with particularly narrow therapeutic ranges. The C_{max} ratio (*see* **Bioavailability**) is allowed to vary more widely than the AUC ratio provided this can be clinically justified. For assessing equivalence of T_{max} (*see* **Bioavailability**), the test statistic is the difference in the values for the test and reference product (Chow SC, Lui JP (1992) *Design and analysis of bioavailability and bioequivalence studies*. Marcel Dekker, New York. Midha KK, Blume HH (eds) (1993) *Bioavailability, bioequivalence and pharmacokinetics*. Medpharm, Stuttgart). Regulatory authorities such as the US Food and Drug Administration (FDA) accept that bioequivalence may sometimes be demonstrated using *in vitro* bioequivalence standard, especially when such an *in vitro* test has been correlated with human *in vivo* bioavailability data. In other situations, bioequivalence may sometimes be demonstrated through comparative clinical trials or pharmacodynamic studies.

Bioequivalent drug products

The US Food and Drug Administration (FDA) uses this term to describe pharmaceutically equivalent or alternative products that display comparable bioavailability when studied under similar experimental conditions. In particular, (a) the rate and extent of absorption of the test drug do not show a significant difference from those of the reference product when administered at the same molar dose of the therapeutic ingredient under similar experimental conditions in either a single dose or multiple doses; or (b) the extent of absorption of the test product does not show a significant difference from the extent of absorption of the reference product when administered at the same molar dose of the therapeutic ingredient under similar experimental conditions in either a single dose or multiple doses and the difference from the reference product in the rate of absorption is intentional, is reflected in its proposed labelling, is not essential to the attainment of effective body drug concentrations on chronic use and is considered medically insignificant for the drug.

When the above are not applicable (e.g. for drug products that are not intended to be absorbed into the bloodstream), other *in vivo* or *in vitro* tests of bioequivalence may be appropriate.

Biological efficacy test (see under Intention to treat analysis)

Biometrics

Biometrics refers to statistical sciences applied to the study of biological phenomena. The term can be used synonymously with **biostatistics.**

Biostatistics

Biostatistics refers to statistical sciences applied to the study of biological phenomena. The term is used synonymously with **biometrics** and increasingly with **medical statistics.**

Blocking

In the design of experiments, blocking is an approach which can be used to eliminate the effect of a factor which is known to influence the result but whose effect is not of direct interest. For example, if an experiment cannot be completed in one day and day-to-day variation is known to affect the result, the experiment can be divided using day as a block factor. The block or day effect can then be eliminated before computation of the model. This reduces noise and enables the effects of other factors to be estimated with greater precision (Maxwell SE, Delaney HD (1990) *Designing experiments and analysing data*. Wadsworth, Belmont, California).

Bootstrapping

Bootstrapping is a computer-based approach for assigning measures of accuracy to statistical estimates. The method is non-parametric in that it does not assume anything about the underlying probability distribution. The idea behind bootstrapping is elegantly simple. Consider some population of size n about which we wish to make some inference.

Let $X = (x_1, x_2, x_3,..., n)$ represent the data points and suppose that we wanted to estimate the standard error of the median. We can draw a bootstrap sample of the same size from X by sampling one point with replacement and repeating this n times. For example, with $n = 6$, we might obtain a bootstrap sample $(x_1, x_2, x_3, x_3, x_6, x_6)$. From these points we can calculate a sample standard deviation. We can repeat the process to obtain m bootstrap samples and m standard deviations. The standard deviation of those sample standard deviations will then give us a bootstrap estimate of the standard error of the median (Efron B, Tibshirani RJ (1993) *An introduction to the bootstrap*. Chapman and Hall, London).

Boundary approach

This is an approach to running and analysing sequential trials whereby a statistic describing the cumulative difference between treatments is plotted against a statistic describing the cumulative amount of evidence. The trial is stopped if one of the pre-specified boundaries is crossed (Whitehead J (1992) *The design and analysis of sequential trials*. 2nd edn. Ellis Horwood, Chichester).

C

CANDA

CANDA is the abbreviation used for computer-assisted new drug application, a procedure which was introduced by the FDA recently (*see* **Prescription Drug User Fee Act 1992**) to speed up the review process of licensing of new drugs.

Carstairs score (*see under* Cluster sampling)

Case-control study

In the study of rare events, for example rare adverse drug reactions, it is usually not possible to mount a controlled study to investigate causation. Impossibly large numbers of subjects would have to be recruited and studied under controlled conditions. Under such circumstances observational studies are used. One of the most powerful designs for such studies, albeit not ideal because of the poor control investigators have over confounding factors, is the case-control design. Cases or subjects with the event of interest (e.g. women of childbearing age and with a stroke) are recruited along with matched control subjects without the event and their history of exposures to various putative risk and confounding factors detailed to identify any significant associations.

Case-control studies are normally classified as retrospective studies in that subjects with a particular event (e.g. a stroke) are identified and their history of exposure to various putative risk factors established retrospectively and compared with that of control subjects. Case-control studies leading to the establishment of a link between phaecomelia in newborns and ingestion of thalidomide by their mothers is an example. The cases were already known and the drug history of their mothers and that of control mothers followed retrospectively. It would clearly not have been ethical to undertake a controlled study to establish the causal association. The adverse effect was not previously seen and was disastrous. In other types of adverse effects, for example pulmonary hypertension, case ascertainment may be difficult and a prospective case-control study may then be undertaken. In such a study, cases are identified prospectively but their exposure history to any association between a risk factor (e.g. anorectic agents) and the adverse event (e.g. pulmonary hypertension) is undertaken retrospectively.

Case fatality rate

The case fatality rate is the rate of death in patients with a particular disease, usually expressed as a percentage (deaths attributed to the disease divided by number of cases of the disease × 100). This rate gives an indication of how deadly a disease is. For example, the case fatality rate for Ebola virus infection is very high while for the influenza virus, it is low except among the elderly. For disease of short duration, the numerators and denominators refer to the same cases. However, with diseases of longer duration, this may not be the case and the measure is no longer a rate but a ratio. For this reason, for diseases such as cancer, the deaths to cases ratio is often quoted instead of case fatality rate. Alternatively, other measures such as five-year survival rates are used. Typically, a group of patients with the same disease is randomized to receive one of the treatments being compared and the percentage of survivors at the end of five years in each subgroup is calculated.

Case management

Case management is the systematic identification and follow-up of high-cost patients so that their care can be co-ordinated through the development of treatment plans to ensure optimum outcome. By definition, cost-effectiveness is an important aspect of case management (*see also* **critical pathway** and Delaney C, Aquilina D (1987) Case management: meeting the challenge of high cost illness. *Employee Benefits Journal.* **12**: 2–8).

Case mix group

Case mix groups are groups of patients who are similar in type and consume the same amount of health care resources when expressed as patient-days of care.

Categorical variable

A variable for which there is only a limited number of possible values and for which there is no logical basis for ordering (e.g. ethnic origin). Alternative names are nominal, polytomous or discrete categorical variable.

Causal relationship

In observational studies, the investigator has no control over the factors which may influence a particular outcome and therefore erroneous causal associations may be inferred. To reduce this risk, Bradford Hill has suggested a number of features which should be carefully considered when assessing the causation of a disease: (i) the strength of association; (ii) consistency in the data (in other words, do all or most of the published studies point in the same direction?); (iii) specificity; (iv) temporal relationship, i.e. exposure to putative factor must precede onset of disease; (v) biological gradient or dose-response relationship; (vi) biological plausibility. It is important to note, however, that biological plausibility depends on the state of knowledge of the day (Hill AB, Hill ID (1991) *Bradford Hill's principles of medical statistics*. 12th edn. Edward Arnold, London).

Cause-specific rate (see Specific rate)

CBA (see Cost benefit analysis)

CEA (see Cost-effectiveness analysis)

Ceiling effect

A ceiling effect is said to occur when a high proportion of subjects in a study have maximum scores on the observed variable. This makes discrimination between subjects at the top end of the scale impossible. For example, an examination paper may lead to, say, 50% of the students scoring 100%. While such a paper may serve as a useful threshold test, it does not allow ranking of the top performers. For this reason, examination of test results for a possible ceiling effect, and the converse floor effect, is often built into the validation of instruments such as those used for measuring quality of life.

Censoring

Censoring is a phenomenon often seen in the analysis of **survival data** or **event history analyses.** To illustrate, consider the follow-up of two groups of terminally ill patients in a comparative study of a new drug and the standard drug. Unfortunately, because we do not have curative drugs for most cancers, time to death is often used as an outcome measure in such studies. If the study lasts for, say, five years, there will be some patients who will survive for longer than this time period and, indeed, our objective is to see how many more patients will fall into this category with the new drug. All we can say of those patients who are still alive at the five-year observation point is that their survival is at least five years. We have no data on how much longer they will live. In other words, their data are censored. Censoring also occurs when patients drop out of studies and are lost to follow-up without the event of interest being observed. Unless the method used for analysis takes account of censoring, we shall end up with biased or imprecise estimates of effect.

Central Statistical Office

The UK Central Statistical Office formed part of the Government Statistical Service but in 1996 it was merged with the Office of Population Census and Surveys to form the Office of National Statistics.

Centre points

In the design of experiments, centre points refer to experimental runs in which all the numerical factors are set at the midpoint of the high and low settings.

Chalmers, TC (1917–95)

An epidemiologist who did much to lay the foundation for evidence-based medicine. He is particularly noted for challenging the notion 'that you can learn how patients should be treated by observing how doctors are treating them'. In his view, the observational approach is rather limited in value and the randomized controlled trial should be regarded as the gold standard in the evaluation of the efficacy of health care interventions. One of his major papers, published in 1992, demonstrated the unreliability of textbook expert recommendations through a cumulative *a*-analysis of controlled trials in myocardial infarction (Lau J, Antman EM, Jimenez-Silva J *et al.* (1992) Cumulative *a*-analysis of therapeutic trials for myocardial intervention. *New England Journal of Medicine.* **327**: 248–54).

Channelling bias

Channelling bias is a term used in pharmacoepidemiological studies to describe the allocation bias which may arise when promotional literature creates in physicians' minds a particular patient profile for a product. For example, if a new non-steroidal drug is promoted as being gentle on the gastrointestinal (GI) tract, physicians may channel patients who they think are at increased risk of GI adverse effects to receive that drug instead of the control drug(s) (Petri H, Urquhart J (1991) Channelling bias in the interpretation of drug effects. *Statistics in Medicine*. **10**: 577–81).

Clinical algorithms
Clinical algorithms are instructions relating to the management of clinical issues, which are organized on the basis of conditional, branching logic (Schoenbaum SC (ed.) (1995) *Using clinical practice guidelines to evaluate quality of care*. V1. US Department of Health and Human Services, Bethesda, MD).

Clinical decision analysis (see Decision analysis)

Clinical effectiveness (see under Effectiveness)

Clinical informatics
Clinical informatics is the subset of medical informatics dealing with clinical practice. The demarcation between the two is not always clear except that the latter is broader and extends to such areas as medical billing and health insurance systems. Practitioners, researchers and students of clinical informatics study such things as (i) the hardware and software used in medical information processing; (ii) the nature of medical data; (iii) the language used in clinical medicine to convey data and knowledge; (iv) medical reasoning; (v) medical computerized expert systems; (vi) medical databases; (vii) medical decision making; (viii) telemedicine; (ix) computer-based training.

Clinical pathway
Clinical pathways are interlinked **clinical practice guidelines** which organize, sequence and time the care given to a typical uncomplicated patient (Pearson SD, Goulart-Fisher D, Lee TiH (1995) Critical pathways as a strategy for improving care: problems and potential. *Annals of Internal Medicine*. **123**: 941–8). The term is also used synonymously with 'critical pathways'.

Clinical phase
The clinical phase in the development of a therapeutic drug refers to the interval from submission of an investigational new drug (IND) application for a new chemical entity (NCE) to submission of a new drug licence application (NDA).

Clinical practice guidelines
Clinical practice guidelines are systematically developed statements to help clinicians and patients to make rational decisions about the most appropriate health care for specific clinical circumstances. Information that one would expect from such guidelines includes: (i) a statement of objective including the targeted health problem and the main reasons for developing recommendations concerning the problem being addressed; (ii) the practice options that were considered; (iii) the main clinical and economic consequences identified as potential outcomes; (iv) the evidence used, including the methods used for systematically collecting the information and its synthesis; (v) the persons and methods used for assigning utilities or values to the potential outcomes; (vi) the benefits, harm and costs that are expected to result from implementation of the guidelines; (vii) methods used to validate the guidelines such as external review and auditing; (viii) identification of sponsors to make explicit any potential conflict of interest; (ix) date of the latest revision of the guideline (Committee to Advise the Public Health Service on Clinical Practice Guidelines. Institute of Medicine. Field MJ, Lohr KN (eds) (1990) *Clinical practice guidelines: directions for a new program.* National Academy Press, Washington DC).

Clinical reasoning
Clinical reasoning refers to the inductive and deductive reasoning which a clinician undertakes when dealing with a patient's health problem. The reasoning is based on clinical experience, tradition, education and intuition. However, there is increasing recognition that these have to be supplemented with quantitative diagnostic reasoning for optimum outcome. For this reason, clinical reasoning is now often broken down into discrete steps for the purpose of research: (i) history taking and physical examination leading to tentative diagnoses; (ii) ordering of appropriate diagnostic tests to provide additional data; (iii) integration of clinical and diagnostic test data; (iv) evaluation of alternative course of action; (v) incorporation of patient preferences in the selection of the most appropriate course of action (Goldman L (1991) Quantitative aspects of clinical reasoning. In: Wilson

JD, Braunwald E, Isselbacher KJ *et al.* (eds) *Harrison's principles of internal medicine.* McGraw-Hill, New York).

Clinical trial

A clinical trial can be defined as any study undertaken to evaluate the clinical effects of an intervention on humans or animals. The control under which such studies are undertaken varies. For estimating efficacy of an intervention, the double-blind, randomized, controlled trial (double-blind RCT) is generally regarded as being the gold standard. In such a trial, one intervention is compared against another, which may be a placebo, to provide a control. Neither the investigator nor the subjects know which treatment is being assigned to whom (i.e. both are blinded) and the assignments are randomized (i.e. subjects are assigned using a validated randomization method). In some instances, it may not be possible for practical or ethical reasons to blind the subjects and/or the investigators (e.g. surgical interventions) and open trials are then resorted to. Randomization may also be on the basis of non-validated allocation schemes such as alternate patient assignments. Such allocations are referred to as quasi-randomization in recognition of the fact that they are less robust. In interpreting the results of clinical trials, it is therefore important to critically assess the designs used. Recently, recommendations have been made on the reporting of clinical trials to ensure that readers have all the information to hand to make a critical appraisal (*see* **CONSORT statement**).

Clinimetrics

Clinimetrics is a term proposed by AR Feinstein to define 'the domain concerned with indexes, rating scales, and other expressions that are used to describe or measure symptoms, physical signs and other distinctly clinical phenomena in clinical medicine (Feinstein AR (1987) *Clinimetrics.* Yale University Press, New Haven). The term is regarded as being synonymous with clinical outcomes research by some authors.

Cluster randomization

A cluster randomized study is one in which a group of subjects is randomized to the same treatment together. An example is when children in some schools are given one vaccine and those of other schools given another and the protection offered compared. The essential feature of studies with cluster randomization is that the unit of analysis is the experimental unit (school, in this case). In analysing such studies, a common approach is to construct a summary statistic for each cluster (school) and then analyse these summary values (Bland JM, Kerry SM (1997) Statistics notes. Trials randomised in clusters. *BMJ*. **315**: 600. Kerry SM, Bland JM (1997) Analysis of a trial randomised in clusters. *BMJ*. **316**: 54).

Cluster sampling

In cluster sampling members of the population to be sampled are first arranged into groups or clusters. The clusters are sampled and those selected are subsampled. Such cluster sampling is often multistaged. A recent study is illustrative. The investigators wanted to draw a sample of 12–17-year-olds from the Community Health Index (a listing of names and addresses of people registered with general practitioners within their health board). The sampling frame consisted of all postcode sectors. Thirty sectors were sampled. These sectors were stratified according to district and Carstairs score (a measure of affluence or deprivation within an area) and a sample of 40 people aged 12–17 years inclusive was drawn from each using a random procedure stratified by age and sex (Hughes K, McKintosh AM, Hastings G *et al.* (1997) Young people, alcohol and designer drinks: quantitative and qualitative study. *BMJ*. **314**: 44–8).

CMA (see Cost minimization analysis)

Cochrane, Archie (1909–88)

A visionary Scottish physician whose criticism of the medical profession for not organizing 'a critical summary, by specialty or subspecialty, adapted periodically, of all relevant randomized trials' to guide practice acted as a catalyst for the establishment of the **Cochrane Collaboration** (*see* Cochrane A, Blythe M (1989) *One man's medicine. An autobiography of Professor Archie Cochrane.* BMA, London).

Cochrane Collaboration

A collaborative network focusing on undertaking and making accessible systematic up-to-date reviews of randomized controlled trials of health care. The collaboration is named after **Archie Cochrane**, a Scottish physician. Initial funding was provided by the UK Department of Health to set up the UK Cochrane Centre but the collaboration is now international with a number of national and regional centres co-ordinating the work of collaborative review groups and networks within their regions. The main output of the collaboration is the **Cochrane Library,** which includes a regularly updated compilation of systematic reviews. Further information may be obtained from their website (*see also* Chalmers I, Altman DG (1995) *Systematic reviews.* BMJ Publishing, London).

Cochrane Library

The Cochrane Library is a quarterly publication (disk/CD-ROM) produced by the **Cochrane Collaboration**. It contains four databases: (i) the Cochrane Database of Systematic Reviews; (ii) the York Database of Reviews of Effectiveness (DARE); (iii) the Cochrane Controlled Trials Register; (iv) the Cochrane Review Methodology Database (CRMD). For further information, contact http://www.cochrane.co.uk.

Coefficient of variation

The coefficient of variation (*CV*) is a measure of residual variation of a set of data expressed as a percentage of the mean. It is defined as follows:

$$CV = (\frac{SD}{Mean}) \times (100)$$

where *SD* is the standard deviation, estimated by the square root of the mean square error.

$$SD = \sqrt{\frac{1}{n-1} \sum_{i=1}^{n} (x_i - \bar{x})^2}$$

where $x_1, x_2, ... x_n$ are the *n* sample observations and $\bar{x}$ is the sample mean.

Cognitive continuum

The cognitive continuum is a theoretical representation of cognitive processing. At one end of the spectrum is highly intuitive thinking and at the other end highly analytical thinking. In between is a mixture of both intuitive and analytical thinking which is characteristic of most of everyday cognitive processing (Figure 3) (Hammond KR, McClelland G, Mumpower J (1980) *Human judgment and decision making: theories, methods and procedures.* Praeger Scientific, New York).

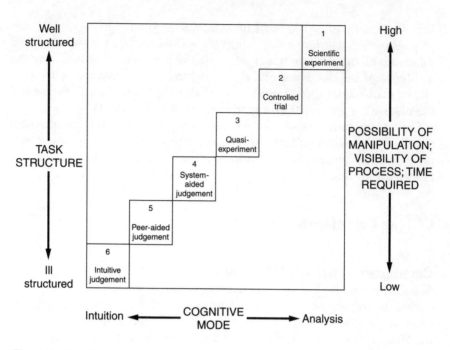

Figure 3 Cognitive continuum

Cohort

In epidemiological studies, the term was originally used to define a group of individuals born during a specified period of time. However, over recent years a looser definition has become common and the term is used to refer to any pre-defined group of people subjected to follow-up (Sartwell PE (1976) Cohorts: the debasement of a word. *American Journal of Epidemiology.* **103**: 536).

Cohort analysis

In a cohort analysis, people of a given, restricted age group are followed prospectively (forward in time) and their rates of disease or death are measured in successive time intervals as they age. Note the restricted definition of cohort used here.

Cohort study

A cohort study is a type of prospective observational study often employed for investigating risk. A typical study may involve recruiting an initially healthy group (cohort) of individuals exposed to different levels of a suspected risk factor (smoking) for a disease (e.g. lung cancer) and following them for a number of years after recruitment. By comparing the incidence of the disease in the different groups, quantitative statements can be made about the strength of association between the risk factor and the disease (*see also under* **Prospective case-control studies**).

Cohort studies have also been referred to as prospective studies (although any study in which subjects are followed forward in time is accurately described as prospective), incidence studies, longitudinal studies or follow-up studies.

COI (see Cost of illness analysis)

Committee on Safety of Medicines

The Committee on Safety of Medicines (CSM) is an advisory body consisting of drug experts, set up to advise the UK ministers of health (the Licensing Authority) on drug licensing. Drug licence applications sent to the Medicines Control Agency are evaluated by its secretariat and recommendations about granting of the licences made with the advice of the CSM. The latter also advises on licence applications which are sent to the European Medicines Evaluation Agency (EMEA) for Europe-wide approval. For such applications, one of the EU member countries acts as rapporteur to co-ordinate all the responses. The CSM also produces a regular leaflet on current problems in pharmacovigilance (http://www.open.gov.uk/mca/).

Community health councils

Community health councils are independent bodies first set up in 1974 by the UK government to represent the interests of the public in the health service in their area.

Community Health Index (see under Cluster sampling)

Compliance

Medicine compliance raises highly complex issues and for this reason there is no consensus on its definition. However, a common working definition is 'the extent to which patients adhere to the advice given by the health care provider'. The term 'adhere' is now generally preferred to 'comply' in defining medication compliance and, indeed, some authors suggest that the term 'medicine compliance' should be replaced by 'medicine adherence' to acknowledge the fact that medical management of a disease should involve active collaboration between patient and health professional. Note that the above definition does not exclude the possibility of intelligent non-compliance being potentially beneficial to patients.

In the study of drug interventions, the percentage of prescribed medication taken by the patient is often used as a possible objective index of medication compliance. This in turn may be used for investigating the impact of non-compliance in pharmacoeconomic studies (Rogers PG, Bullman WR (1995) *Prescription medicine compliance: a review of baseline knowledge.* National Council on Patient Information and Education, Washington).

More recently, in the medical literature, the term 'compliance' has also been used to define the extent to which prescribers adhere to consensus treatment guidelines.

Comprehensive cohort study

In many types of trials, such as in breast cancer trials involving surgery or coronary artery trials, only a small proportion of the patients who are approached consent to randomization and therefore recruiting sufficient numbers of patients to the trials is very hard. The comprehensive cohort study attempts to overcome this problem by considering the patients who agree to randomization as a subgroup of a larger cohort which includes those who refuse. With proper analysis, it is argued that reliable estimates of comparative efficacy can be obtained. Unlike post-randomization consent trials, patients are randomized in the normal way and less bias is likely to be introduced. The method is not universally accepted (Olscheski M, Scheurlen H (1985) Comprehensive cohort study: an alternative to randomized consent design in a breast preservation trial. *Methods of Information in Medicine.* **24**: 131–4).

Confidence interval

A range of values, calculated from sample observations, to contain the true parameter value with a known probability. Thus, a 95% confidence interval is one which, when estimated repeatedly, will 95% of the time be expected to include the true value of the parameter being estimated. The probability estimate refers to the interval (a random variable) and not to the parameter which is regarded as being fixed (*see* **Credible interval**). Most journals now require that confidence intervals be attached to point estimates of parameters cited in reports submitted to them, to give readers an indication of the precision of those estimates (Li Wan Po A (1998) *Statistics for pharmacists.* Blackwell Science, Oxford).

Confounder

A confounder is a variable which is correlated with the response of interest in a clinical trial or in an epidemiological study. Confounders may lead to erroneous conclusions being drawn, particularly in observational studies. For example, prior to the identification of micro-organisms, various spurious explanations were put forward for infectious disease. Acne was at one time blamed on excessive masturbation!

Confounding by indication

Confounding by indication is the bias which may arise in observational studies when patients with the worst prognoses are allocated preferentially to one treatment. Since randomization is not used, patients treated with one drug may be systematically different from those treated with the other. For example, in a recent observational study it was claimed that use of antihypertensives in the elderly was associated with a higher incidence of myocardial infarction (Grobbee DE, Hoes AW (1997) Confounding and indication for treatment in evaluation of drug treatment for hypertension. *BMJ.* **315**: 1151–4).

Conjoint analysis

Conjoint analysis is a multivariate statistical method for deriving utilities to represent respondents' preferences for product attributes. The method attempts to identify trade-offs which the respondents are willing to make with respect to the various product attributes. From the results, objective decisions can then be made about preferred combinations of attributes for products or services to be developed. Conjoint analysis is now widely used in marketing research for the purpose of pricing, new product/ concept identification, market segmentation, competitive analysis and product repositioning (Hair JF Jr, Anderson RE, Tatham RL, Black WC (1995) *Multivariate data analysis.* 4th edn. Prentice Hall, Englewood Cliffs).

Consensus development conferences

These are run by the US National Institutes of Health (NIH) to elicit consensus statements about particular health care interventions. At these conferences, multidisciplinary experts are asked to examine the evidence on the particular issue at hand to come up with a consensus view, typically within two days. In some cases, the panel may arrange to meet prior to the conference to determine what information is needed and to assess written material. Recent conferences have considered subjects such as breast cancer screening (Fletcher SW (1997) Whither scientific deliberation in health policy deliberations? *New England Journal of Medicine*. **336**: 1180–3).

CONSORT statement

A statement on the quality of reporting of clinical trials, prepared by a group of journal editors and clinical trialists (*see under* **Clinical trials**). The recommendations are shown below.

Title Identify the study as a randomized trial

Abstract Use a structured abstract

Method *Protocol* Describe:

(i) planned study population and inclusion and exclusion criteria

(ii) planned interventions and their timing

(iii) primary and secondary outcome measures and the minimum important difference and indicate how the target sample size was projected

(iv) rationale and methods for statistical analyses, detailing main comparative analyses and whether they were completed on an intention-to-treat basis

(v) prospectively defined stopping rules, if warranted.

Assignment Describe:

(i) unit of randomization (e.g. individual, cluster, geographic)

(ii) method used to generate allocation schedule

(iii) method of allocation concealment and timing of assignment

(iv) method to separate the generator from the executor of assignment.

Masking (blinding)   Describe:

(i) mechanism (e.g. capsules, tablets)

(ii) similarity of treatment characteristics (e.g. appearance, taste)

(iii) allocation schedule control (location of code during trial and when broken)

(iv) evidence for successful blinding among participants, persons doing intervention, outcome assessors, and data analysts.

Results   *Participants*   Provide a trial profile (Figure 4) summarizing participant flow and number and timing of randomization assignment, intervention follow-up measurements for each randomized group.

Analysis   (i) State estimated effect of intervention on primary and secondary outcome measures, including point estimates and measures of precision (confidence interval).

(ii) State results in absolute numbers when feasible (e.g. 10/20, not 50%).

(iii) Present summary data and appropriate descriptive and inferential statistics in sufficient detail to permit alternative analyses and replication.

(iv) Describe prognostic variables by treatment group and any attempt to adjust for them.

(v) Describe protocol violations from the study as planned, together with the reasons.

Discussion   (i) State specific interpretation of study findings, including sources of bias and imprecision (internal validity) and discussion of external validity, including appropriate quantitative measures when possible.

(ii) State general interpretation of the data in light of totality of the available evidence.

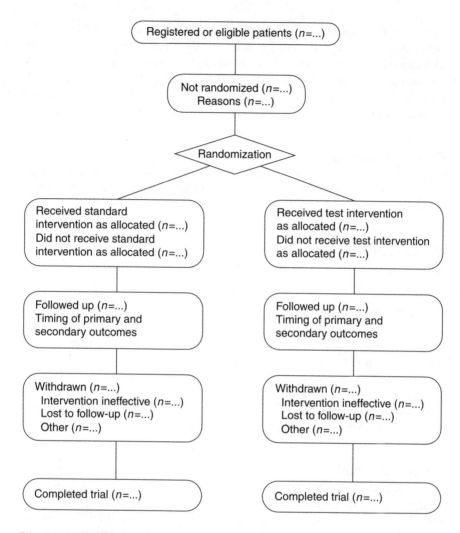

Figure 4 CONSORT statement: CONSORT trial profile

(Begg C, Cho M, Eastwood S *et al.* (1996) Improving the quality of reporting of randomized controlled trials: the CONSORT statement. *Journal of the American Medical Association.* **276**: 637–9).

Construct

A construct is a variable constructed through informed scientific theory. Such a variable is abstract and latent rather than concrete and observable.

Nearly all theories in psychology refer to constructs rather than to specific behaviours (Nunnally JC, Bernstein IH (1994) *Psychometric theory*. 3rd edn. McGraw-Hill, New York). Anxiety and intelligence are examples of constructs. We cannot measure these directly but have to use surrogate measures such as the intelligence quotient (IQ) test, with all the associated problems of validity which such an approach brings about.

Consumer surplus

Consumer surplus refers to the difference between what a consumer actually pays for a good or service and the most that he or she would be willing to pay.

Contestable market

A contestable market is one in which there are no entry and exit barriers.

Context effect

It is being increasingly recognized that patients' responses to treatments may be affected by various factors such as how the investigator presents the interventions. These non-specific effects are referred to as context effects. To neutralize such effects, randomization, concealed assignment of treatment and blinding are used in well-conducted trials. The term 'context effect' has also been suggested as a better way of describing the 'placebo effect', as the latter has derogatory connotations.

Contingency table

A contingency table is one in which subjects or objects from a group are assigned to mutually exclusive categories or cells. In other words, each individual is entered in one cell only. Each cell gives the total number (or counts) of subjects or objects belonging to a subgroup. An example of a contingency table is shown in Table 1.

Table I Contingency table showing hypothetical data from a comparative trial of three drugs on mortality. Each arm of the study entered 100 patients

Drug	Deaths	Survived	Total
Drug A	5	95	100
Drug B	20	80	100
Placebo	40	60	100
Total	65	235	300

The contingency table shown is a 3 row × 2 column table and is usually referred to simply as a 3 × 2 table; 2 × 2 tables are particularly commonly encountered. Multidimensional contingency tables are widely used in advanced categorical data analyses but require advanced graphical multivariate methods for representation on paper.

Contingent valuation

Estimates of **willingness to pay** for goods for which there is no market can be obtained using survey methods. Individuals are asked how much they would be willing to pay to avoid or overcome a certain state (e.g. avoidance of a particular morbidity). Using such an approach, sometimes referred to as 'contingent valuation' or **expressed preference**, the questions can be either open-ended or binary (Figure 5). In the former, the patient is asked the maximum amount he or she would be prepared to pay for the current treatment in a face-to-face or telephone interview or questionnaire. In order to improve response rate, response aids such as a bidding game are used. The patient is shown a value which is either rejected or accepted. The value is then altered until the maximum payment which is acceptable to the patient is identified. Alternatively, the patient may be shown a range of payment values from which a choice is made. The open-ended approach

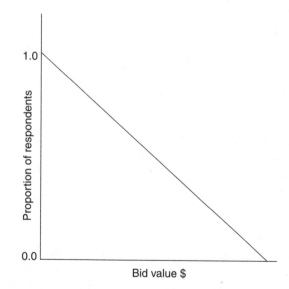

Figure 5 Contingent valuation: The calculation of willingness to pay using the binary contingent valuation method

is subject to starting point bias and because of this the binary contingent valuation method is becoming more popular. With this method, each respondent is asked to accept or reject a single bid or payment which will have to be paid in exchange for the treatment being evaluated. A patient who accepts the bid is assumed to have a maximum willingness to pay in excess of that amount. Conversely, one who rejects the bid is assumed to have a maximum willingness to pay which is lower. By stratifying a sample of respondents and presenting the same bid to each member of a given stratum, it is therefore possible to estimate the proportion of individuals who would be willing to pay each bid. A graph of bid value ($) against proportion of respondents willing to pay can then be drawn. The mean willingness to pay is obtained by estimating the area under the curve using appropriate statistical methods. Using these methods, it is possible to take account of variables such as income or educational level which may affect willingness to pay. The binary approach is sometimes referred to as a closed-ended method which is considered separately from the contingent valuation method (Mitchell RC, Carson RT (1989) *Using surveys to value public goods: resources for the future.* Washington DC. Johannsson P-O (1995) *Evaluating health risks.* Cambridge University Press, Cambridge).

Continuous variable

A variable which can take an infinite number of values (e.g. height and weight) within a range. In practice, statisticians often treat variables with more than about ten values as continuous.

Contract curve (see under Efficiency)

Convenience sample

A convenience sample is made up of individuals or groups selected by the investigator because they were convenient at the time or location of sampling.

Cost

The cost of a product or service can be defined as the monetary value of the resources consumed in its production or delivery. Such costs can be subdivided into direct costs, which involve actual transfer of money, and indirect costs, which represent resources committed but unpaid. Some types of resources are required to be committed irrespective of level of output within given ranges. For example, a tabletting machine is required for producing tablets irrespective of whether the output is 5000 or 500 000 per day until the capacity of the machine is exceeded. Such costs are called fixed costs. Variable costs, on the other hand, refer to costs which change with output. The cost of drugs and excipients is an example of a variable cost. Similarly, a salary is a fixed cost but sales-related bonuses are variable costs.

Cost is therefore not synonymous with price which is what the customer is asked to pay for a good or service. Price is usually higher than cost to enable the provider to make profits but within health care, the charge for a service often does not fully reflect the resources consumed. Indeed, under many national health care schemes, the charge for many services is zero but clearly the cost is not.

In therapeutic cost-effectiveness analyses, three categories of medical resources are usually costed: (i) resources used by the therapy itself, including any necessary monitoring and resources used to treat adverse effects; (ii) resources used during additional life-years; (iii) resources gained from reduced need for other services as a result of the therapy. In some pharmacoeconomic analyses, cost of transportation, home help and changes in earned income are also included under costs (*see also* **Average cost, Incremental cost** and **Opportunity cost**).

Cost benefit analysis

This is a type of economic assessment in which both costs and benefits are expressed in monetary terms to provide a cost:benefit ratio. The fact that, in this type of analysis, everything is expressed in monetary terms makes it possible to compare disparate interventions. However, this requirement is also a constraint since outcomes of medical interventions are often difficult to value, being dependent on the patients' individual perspectives.

Cost:benefit ratio

This is the ratio given by dividing the total cost of a programme or intervention by the benefits expressed as savings in projected expenditure.

Cost-effective

A number of meanings are attached to the term 'cost-effective' when used colloquially. Some use the term synonymously with 'effective' while others attach the notion of cost saving to it. In pharmacoeconomic analysis, it is suggested that the term be used to describe a strategy or treatment when it is (i) less costly and at least as effective; (ii) more costly and more effective but the added efficacy is worth paying for at the price offered; (iii) less effective and less costly but the additional cost of the alternative is too high for the added benefits provided (Doubilet P, Weinstein MC, McNeil BJ (1986) Use and misuse of the term 'cost-effective' in medicine. *New England Journal of Medicine.* **314**: 253–6).

Cost-effectiveness analysis (CEA)

This is a type of economic assessment in which interventions having a common outcome (e.g. lives saved, life-years gained or reduction in number of epileptic fits) are compared. CEA is widely used for comparing drug efficacy (e.g. anti-ulcer drugs with benefits expressed as ulcers cured). The results of a CEA are expressed as a cost-effectiveness ratio (e.g. $ per ulcer prevented). The term is also commonly used more generically to refer to any cost gain analysis.

Cost-effectiveness ratio

This is the ratio of total cost of an intervention divided by the gain in selected health outcome (e.g. cost per myocardial infarction prevented or cost per life-year gained). Note that although the term is referred to as a ratio, it is not usually dimensionless.

Cost of illness analysis (COI)

Cost of illness analyses (also called burden of illness analyses) are economic studies aimed at estimating the economic burden of a particular disease. COI analyses have, for example, been undertaken for smoking-related diseases, iatrogenic disease and psoriasis. Pharmaceutical manufacturers often undertake cost of illness studies in order to make projections about savings in health care costs arising from wider use of their drugs. Policy makers use results from COI studies when assigning health care priorities.

Cost minimization analysis (CMA)

In economic analysis, CMA is used when the interventions to be compared can be assumed to produce equal benefits. The aim then is to determine which intervention is associated with the least (minimum) cost. In pharmacoeconomic analyses, CMA may be used for comparing clinically equivalent generic products (generics).

Cost utility analysis (CUA)

In this type of economic assessment, the benefits of intervention (e.g. drug or programme) are measured in utility units or utility-weighted life-years. The results are then expressed in terms of cost per utility unit or per utility-weighted life-year. Perhaps the most widely used measure of utility is the quality-adjusted life-year (QALY).

Cox proportional hazards model

This is one of the most widely used models in **survival analysis**. The regression model relates time to event (e.g. failure, death, etc.) to a set of descriptor variables (e.g. patients' ages or treatment received). The modelling takes account of the whole survival curve, including **censoring**. Descriptor variables can be used as part of the regression model or as stratification factors. In the regression model, the effect of a variable is expressed through its impact on the hazard or instantaneous risk of death at any given time (Cox DR (1972) Regression models and life tables. *Journal of the Royal Statistical Society B series*. **34**: 187–220).

CPT (see Current procedural terminology)

Credibility or credible interval

A credibility interval is the Bayesian version of a confidence interval. Its interpretation is more intuitive than that of the classic **confidence interval** in that it refers to the probability of the parameter of interest being in a pre-assigned interval, conditional on the observed data. For example, if in a study to estimate what proportion (Π) of patients would respond to a new treatment, we observe that a proportion p_1 of a sample of patients responded and report that the associated 95% credibility interval is [a,b], we mean that given the observation p_1, there is a 95% probability of Π being in that interval. The credibility interval is also referred to variously as a (e.g. 95%) posterior probability interval, a (e.g. 95%) highest density region or a (e.g. 95%) Bayesian confidence interval (Lee PM (1989) *Bayesian statistics: an introduction*. Oxford University Press, New York).

Criterion standard (see Gold standard)

Critical incident technique

The critical incident technique is a qualitative research method which is particularly useful when the investigator of a complex issue (e.g. prescribing by general practitioners) wishes to understand the reasons for a particular behaviour (e.g. prescribing a new drug instead of an established one). The method uses factual accounts of actual events in which the purpose and consequences of the behaviour are clear (Bradley CP (1992) Uncomfortable prescribing decisions: a critical incident study. *BMJ*. **304**: 294–6. Fitzpatrick R, Boulton M (1994) Qualitative research methods for assessing health care. *Quality in Health Care*. **3**: 107–13).

Critical literature appraisal

Critical literature appraisal is the application of critical thinking when evaluating the literature. With critical appraisal, the practitioner should be (i) better able to identify reliable and relevant research evidence; (ii) more discriminating in reading; (iii) more consistent in using good quality evidence in decision making; (iv) better able to develop evidence-based services (Milne R, Donald A (1995) Piloting short workshops on the critical appraisal of reviews. *Health Trends*. **27**: 120–3).

Critical pathway

A critical pathway is a pre-determined case management pathway for hospitalized patients from admission to discharge to ensure optimum outcome in a cost-effective way. Check points and systematic records of each patient's progress are integral components of a critical pathway and these allow subsequent auditing of procedures and outcomes. The care given to the typical uncomplicated patient is organized, sequenced and timed. Critical pathways are developed to facilitate seamless multidisciplinary interaction between different health care workers involved in managing the cases concerned (*see* **Case management, Clinical pathway** and Giuliano KK, Poirier CE (1991) Nursing case management: critical pathways to desirable outcomes. *Nursing Management*. **22**: 52–5. Pearson SD, Goulart-Fisher D, Lee TIH (1995) Critical pathways as a strategy for improving care: problems and potential. *Annals of Internal Medicine*. **123**: 941–8).

Critical thinking

Critical thinking is the systematic evaluation of data presented to us. This requires an ability to interact with and question whatever information is presented so that we can reliably defend or revise our initial beliefs. In particular, in the evaluation of an argument, using critical thinking we are encouraged to (i) identify the issues and conclusions presented to us; (ii) identify the assumptions made; (iii) assess the quality of the evidence presented to us; (iv) identify any omissions and fallacies in the arguments; (v) suggest possible alternative explanations; (vi) assess the validity of any conclusions and generalizations made. In essence, the important components of critical thinking are those which are applied when undertaking a systematic overview (Browne MN, Keeley SM (1994) *Asking the right questions: a guide to critical thinking.* 4th edn. Prentice Hall, London).

Cronbach's alpha

A statistic which is used to quantify internal consistency. It takes values in the range −1 to +1. High values are desirable when high internal consistency is required of an instrument, such as when discriminating between different groups. When developing an instrument to have such discriminative properties, Cronbach's alpha may be increased by deleting items which do not correlate highly with the others or introducing others which correlate better (Cronbach LJ (1951) Coefficient alpha and the internal structure of tests. *Psychometrica.* **6**: 297–334). Experts suggest that in the early stages of research, a reliability alpha value of 0.7 is sufficient and seeking values higher than 0.8 may be wasteful of funds. However, when measurements on individuals are being made, a reliability of at least 0.9 should be sought with a target of at least 0.95 (Nunally JC, Bernstein IH (1994) *Psychometric theory.* 3rd edn. McGraw-Hill, New York).

The formula for calculating Cronbach's alpha value α is:

$$\alpha_{kk} = \frac{k}{k-1} \frac{\sigma_y^2 - \sum \sigma_i^2}{\sigma_y^2}$$

where: σ_y^2 = the variance of the total scores

σ_i^2 = variance of the set of 0,1 scores representing correct and incorrect answers on item i

n = number of items.

Cross-design synthesis

In a traditional meta-analysis, results from studies using the same designs are pooled to give a more precise estimate of effect. Typically, only results from randomized controlled trials (RCTs) are pooled although results from observational studies have also been aggregated. It is now generally recognized that while RCTs provide results which are least prone to bias, the results may not be generalizable to the range of relevant patients, treatment implementations and outcome criteria which count in medical practice. The US General Accounting Office (GAO) recently proposed an approach which extends the logic of meta-analysis by combining results from studies that have different, complementary designs so that the strengths of the different designs can be captured while minimizing weaknesses. The four major tasks of this methodology are described as follows by the GAO.

Task I   Assess existing randomized studies for generalizability across the full range of relevant patients.

Task II   Assess database analyses for imbalanced comparison groups.

Task III   Adjust the results of each randomized study and each database analysis, compensating for biases as needed.

Task IV   Synthesize the studies' adjusted results within and across design categories.

One difficulty with this approach is that estimates of bias are difficult to obtain. Some authors have suggested adjustments to the Mann–Whitney statistic (which estimates the probability of a random patient performing better on a test treatment than a random patient on the control treatment) of −0.15 for studies with non-random sequential assignment and −0.11 for non-double blind randomized controlled trials. (United States General Accounting Office (1992) *Report to congressional requesters. Cross-design synthesis. A new synthesis for medical effectiveness research. Report GAO/PEMD-92-18.* Colditz GA, Miller JN, Mosteller F (1989) How study design affects outcome in comparisons of therapy. I: Medical. *Statistics in Medicine.* 8: 441–54.)

Cross-subsidization
Cross-subsidization refers to the way in which the revenues from the profitable parts or aspects of an organization are used to subsidize the inefficient or unprofitable parts or aspects.

Crude death rate
This is simply the number of deaths divided by the population at risk over a specified interval without adjustment or standardization for

demographic characteristics (*see also* **Specific rate**). Crude death rates are therefore misleading when comparing mortality in different countries and age-specific death rates are better in such analyses.

CSO (see Central Statistical Office)

Culyer Report

The Culyer Report is a report to the UK Minister for Health by the Research and Development (R&D) Task Force under the chairmanship of Professor Anthony Culyer. The terms of reference for the Task Force were to consider whether changes in the conduct and support of R&D in and by the NHS should be recommended and to advise on alternative funding and support mechanisms for R&D, including transitional measures, within available resources. A summary of the report can be downloaded from http://www.eoi.bris.ac.uk/rd/aboutus/culyer/cul.htm.

Cumulative meta-analysis (see under Meta-analysis)

Current procedural terminology

Current procedural terminology (CPT) refers to the classification of medical procedures developed under the aegis of the American Medical Association. First published in 1966, it is now in its fourth edition (CPT-4). The latter was used as a basis for developing the Healthcare Common Procedure Coding System (HCPCS) used by the US Health Care Financing Administration which administers Medicare and Medicaid, their two large public health insurance systems (American Medical Association (1994) *Physicians' current procedural terminology: CPT-95.* AMA, Chicago).

D

DEADLE

DEADLE stands for Declining Exponential Approximation of Discounted Life Expectancy. The model approximates life expectancy using an exponential model (*see* **DEALE**) and then discounts the estimated life expectancy (LE) to the present using the formula:

$$LE = \frac{1}{\mu + i}$$

where μ is the mortality rate constant and i the effective discount rate. A value of 5% is common but values of 3–6% have been used (Martens L, van Doorslaer E (1990) Dealing with discounting. An application to the cost effectiveness of intracoronary thrombolysis with streptokinase. *International Journal of Technical Assessment in Health Care.* **6**: 139–45).

DEALE

DEALE stands for Declining Exponential Approximation of Life Expectancy, a method developed for approximating life expectancy. The method describes survival probability $P(t)$ as an exponential decay curve:

$$P(t) = e^{-\mu t}$$

where μ = mortality rate constant and t the time. If t is in units of year (y) then μ is in units of y^{-1}. The life expectancy is then estimated by integrating the area under the survival probability time curve. This can be shown to be equal to the reciprocal of the mortality rate constant or μ^{-1}. The expected number of remaining life-years can therefore be compared for groups with different mortality rates by estimating the mortality rate constants from the corresponding survival probability time curves (Beck JR, Kassirer JP, Paulker SG (1982) A convenient approximation of life expectancy: the 'DEALE'. *American Journal of Medicine.* **73**: 863–97).

Deaths to cases ratio (see Case fatality rate)

DEC reports

DEC reports are drug evaluation reports produced by regional drug development and evaluation committees in the United Kingdom. The reports, first published by the Wessex region, provide information about the evidence pertaining to the efficacy, safety and cost-effectiveness of particular interventions. To inject local relevance, issues such as the local prevalence of any clinical conditions being considered and the impact of adoption of particular treatments on regional health care budgets are discussed. Published DEC reports, for example, considered issues such as the use of evening primrose oil in pre-menstrual syndrome and mastalgia and 5-fluorouracil as adjuvant chemotherapy in Dukes stage C colorectal cancer.

Decision analysis

Decision analysis is the scientific study of **decision making**.

Decision making

Decision making is intentional and reflective choice in response to a perceived need and is particularly hard under conditions of uncertainty. Careful structuring of the decision-making process and the systematic evaluation of evidence is necessary for the most rational decisions to be arrived at. It is important to note that the most rational decision will not always yield the best physical or economic outcome. For example, presented with a league table of the cost-effectiveness of various medical interventions (e.g. QALY rankings), a group of decision makers may well adopt a less cost-effective intervention on equity grounds (Teilhard de Chardin P (1959) *The phenomenon of man*. Harper and Brothers, New York. Ubel PA, DeKay ML, Baron J, Asch DA (1996) Cost-effectiveness analysis. *New England Journal of Medicine*. **334**: 1174–7. Hadorn DC (1991) Setting health-care priorities in Oregon: cost-effectiveness meets the rule of rescue. *Journal of the American Medical Association*. **265**: 1294–301).

Decision sciences

Decision sciences describes the field of study concerned with understanding and improving decision making. In addition to addressing issues of methodology relating to how best to solve problems (prescriptive theories), decision scientists also study how decision makers (individuals, groups or organizations) identify problems which need addressing and how they learn from the results of their actions (descriptive theories). The field of decision sciences has its roots in many disciplines, including economics, management science, philosophy, psychology, social science and statistics. Medical decision making, which draws heavily on the clinical sciences as well as the above disciplines, has been the subject of much development over the past three decades (Kleindorfer PR, Kunreuther HC, Schoemaker PJH (1993) *Decision sciences*. Cambridge University Press, Cambridge).

Defined daily dose
The defined daily dose (DDD) is a measure of the standard daily thera- peutic dose. The number of defined daily doses is obtained by dividing the total amount of drug prescribed by the defined daily dose for the drug. For example, the defined daily dose of ranitidine is 300 mg. Therefore, if a practice prescribes 150 000 mg of the drug, this is equivalent to 500 DDDs. The World Health Organization publishes a list of DDDs for various drugs (WHO (1997) *Guidelines for defined daily doses*. WHO, Geneva).

Delphi technique
The Delphi technique is a consensus method for making forecasts. In health care it is often used for making predictions about costs or demands for health care services whenever reliable data for making objective predic- tions are not available. The Delphi technique has, for example, been used for predicting the epidemiology of acquired immune deficiency disease so that health care provisions for such patients can be planned and for pre- dicting the course of progression of hairy cell leukaemia in patients treated with or without interferon (Ozer H, Golomb HM, Zimmerman H, Spiegel RJ (1989) Cost-benefit analysis of interferon Alfa-2b in the treatment of hairy cell leukaemia. *Journal of the National Cancer Institute*. **81**: 594–602).

The Delphi technique is usually classified as a qualitative research method although the predictions being made are usually quantitative. Usually three different types of participants are involved in the Delphi process: (i) decision makers, who are a group of experts who will make the forecast; (ii) staff personnel who will assist in the administration of the project; (iii) expert respondents whose judgements are valued.

Once the three groups have been selected, the following steps take place: (i) development and administration of the first questionnaire; (ii) analysis of the results of the first questionnaire; (iii) development and administration of the second questionnaire and simultaneous feedback of the information to the respondents; (iv) analysis of the results of the second questionnaire and, if necessary, further iteration with more questionnaires until consensus is achieved. Feedback of the information to the respondents at each stage; (v) presentation of the consensus results; (vi) make forecast.

Deterministic models (see Stochastic model)

Discounting
In economic analyses, the fact that costs that are incurred sooner are more keenly felt than those that are incurred later (a phenomenon referred to as 'positive rate of time preference') is taken into account by discounting costs as they accrue over time. Costs of alternative therapies, with different time profiles, can therefore be expressed uniformly in terms of present values. The formula used for discounting is as follows:

$$P = \frac{C_1}{1+r} + \frac{C_2}{(1+r)^2} + \frac{C_3}{(1+r)^3} + \cdots + \frac{C_n}{(1+r)^n}$$

where P = present value, r = discount rate and a value between 3% and 5% is often recommended, $C_1, C_2, C_3, \ldots, C_n$ are the costs in year 1, 2, 3,...,n.

Disease management
Disease management is a systematic population-based approach to identifying those at risk, intervening using the best systematically reviewed evidence and measuring patient outcomes once an intervention is in effect. Important operational aspects include (i) the development of clear clinical guidelines; (ii) agreement on the part of providers and patients to participate; (iii) establishment of an efficient and effective information infrastructure; (iv) well-designed and tested interventions; (v) a logical plan for the collection of outcomes (Epstein RS, McGlynn MG (1997) Disease management. What is it? *Disease Management and Health Outcomes.* 1: 3–10).

Domain
In quality of life assessments, a domain is a range of observables used to measure a particular construct. For example, one can refer to a physical function domain which includes a range of items aimed at defining that

particular construct. Similarly, in scales such as the Short-Form 36 scale, we have domains for constructs such as mental health and social functioning.

Dominance (in economic assessments)

In economic assessments of health care, one is normally concerned with ranking alternative interventions and various types of methods are available (*see* **Cost benefit analysis, Cost-effectiveness analysis, Cost minimization analysis** or **Cost utility analysis**). Irrespective of which method is used, the ranking is based on some cost to benefit ratio.

A dominated alternative is one which is less effective and more costly than another or when its incremental cost-effectiveness ratio is higher than that of the next more effective treatment (Karlsson G, Johannesson M (1996) The decision rules of cost-effectiveness analysis. *Pharmacoeconomics*. **9**: 113–20).

Drug development

The drug development process is a complicated and expensive one. It has been estimated that on average it costs over two hundred million dollars to bring a drug to the market. Figure 6 illustrates the various steps in the process. Studies in humans are often classified into stages. Phase I studies are those undertaken to define the disposition of a new drug in healthy volunteers. Phase II studies are those undertaken in small numbers of patients as pilots for subsequent larger studies and for defining the most appropriate doses. Phase III studies are often referred to as definitive or pivotal efficacy studies as these are undertaken with a view to confirming the efficacy suggested by Phase II studies. One to three thousand patients may be involved. The results of those studies form the basis for marketing licence applications. Since clinical trials on relatively small numbers of subjects are unlikely to reveal rare adverse side-effects, post-marketing (Phase IV) studies are undertaken to identify such problems. Sometimes during wider use of a new drug, it appears that the drug has additional therapeutic effects. New trials (Phase IIIa) are then undertaken to assess these. If confirmed, the drug company concerned can apply to have the indications for the drug widened.

Drug development and evaluation committee reports
(see **DEC reports**)

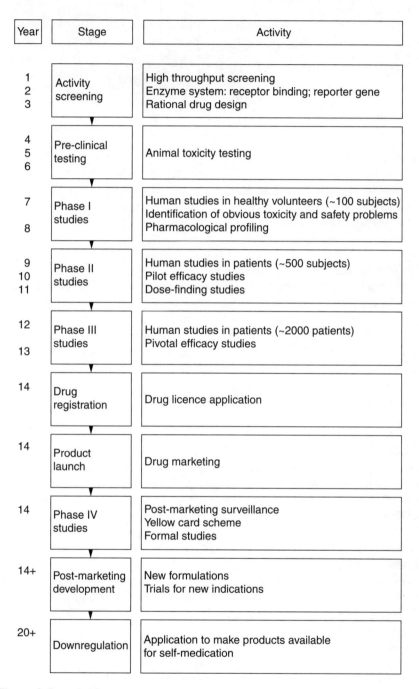

Year	Stage	Activity
1 2 3	Activity screening	High throughput screening Enzyme system: receptor binding; reporter gene Rational drug design
4 5 6	Pre-clinical testing	Animal toxicity testing
7 8	Phase I studies	Human studies in healthy volunteers (~100 subjects) Identification of obvious toxicity and safety problems Pharmacological profiling
9 10 11	Phase II studies	Human studies in patients (~500 subjects) Pilot efficacy studies Dose-finding studies
12 13	Phase III studies	Human studies in patients (~2000 patients) Pivotal efficacy studies
14	Drug registration	Drug licence application
14	Product launch	Drug marketing
14	Phase IV studies	Post-marketing surveillance Yellow card scheme Formal studies
14+	Post-marketing development	New formulations Trials for new indications
20+	Downregulation	Application to make products available for self-medication

Figure 6 Drug development

Ecological fallacy

This term is used to describe a spurious association due to inferring relationships at the individual level from associations between variables at the population level (Robinson WS (1950) Ecological correlations and the behaviour of individuals. *American Sociological Reviews*. **15**: 351–7).

Ecological study

An ecological study is one in which data are collected and correlated at the population level rather than at the level of the individual. The unit of observation in an ecological study is a group of people such as a school, a factory, a city or a nation. An example of an ecological study is the study of the relationship between average sales of beta-agonist inhalers and deaths using data from different countries over the same time interval. Such ecological studies can also be undertaken on the same population at different times.

(The) Economic problem

The problem of allocating scarce resources to meet competing ends is sometimes referred to as the economic problem or the fundamental economic problem. It can be argued that, without scarcity, there is no need for economics as a discipline.

Edgeworth box

The Edgeworth box is a graphical method for describing concepts such as (i) interrelations between two markets; (ii) mutual gains and trade-offs; (iii) Pareto efficiency. Figure 7 shows an Edgeworth box illustrating the concept of Pareto efficiency.

The south-west and north-east corners of the box provide the point of reference co-ordinates for subjects 1 and 2 respectively. The north-west and south-east corners refer to the maximum amount of goods 1 and 2 (i.e. Q1 and Q2) to be traded. The subjects have their own indifference

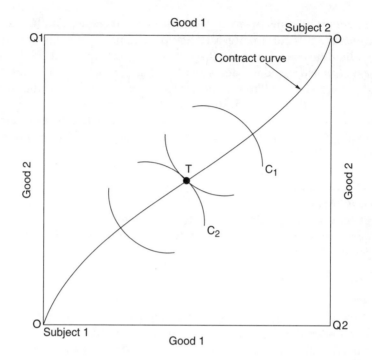

Figure 7 Edgeworth box illustrating the concept of Pareto efficiency

curves showing combinations of goods 1 and 2 which they would be equally happy with (curves C). The point at which two **indifference curves** for the two subjects are at a tangent to each other (point T) is **Pareto efficient** since at that point it is impossible to improve the position of one subject without harming that of the other. Within the Edgeworth box, there will be many points which are **Pareto efficient**. These alternatives fall along what is referred to as the **contract curve** for the two subjects (Folland S, Goodman AC, Stano M (1997) *The economics of health and health care*. 2nd edn. Prentice Hall, New Jersey).

Educational outreach (see Academic detailing)

Effect size

In meta-analysis, effect size refers to the standardized effect observed. By standardizing the effect, the result becomes dimensionless so that the pooling of effects obtained with different measurement scales can be undertaken. While this overcomes one problem, it creates another because the results are difficult to interpret. Standardizing the effect is undertaken by dividing the estimate of effect by the control group standard deviation (s_c) or the pooled standard deviation (s_p). The former is sometimes called Glass's effect size and the latter Hedge's effect size, after the authors who proposed them. In reporting effect sizes, it is important to make explicit whether the pooled or control standard deviation is used (Hedges LV, Olkin I (1985) *Statistical methods for meta-analysis*. Academic Press, San Diego).

Effectiveness
The effectiveness of a drug refers to the extent to which it achieves its intended purpose for the broad range of patients who will receive it in practice (*see* **Efficacy**).

Efficacy
The efficacy of a drug refers to the extent to which it achieves its intended purpose under the strict conditions of randomized controlled trials, in patients typically recruited in such trials (*see* **Effectiveness**).

Efficacy analysis (*see under* Intention to treat analysis)

Efficiency
In the pharmacoeconomic literature, two types of efficiency are often referred to: **technical efficiency** and **allocative efficiency**. With technical efficiency, one is concerned with the technical performance of interventions for dealing with the same problem (e.g. management of prostate cancer) while with allocative efficiency, the focus is on how best to allocate scarce resources across different competing objectives (e.g. provision of day care services versus the setting up of a breast screening clinic). The latter is regarded as being a higher form of efficiency than the former and requires value judgements to be made about the relative value of pursuing different objectives and hence different outputs.

More generally, in economics, efficiency refers to optimum use of resources. Technical efficiency is achieved when the maximum amount of output is generated from a given amount of resources. An old hospital was not technically efficient if a new one brings about a reduction in costs for the same throughput of patients. On the other hand, optimum allocative efficiency occurs when it is not possible to reallocate resources to make one person better off without also making another worse off. An improvement in allocative efficiency is achieved if production costs are reduced to allow a lower selling price for a medicine. Consumers are better off and manufacturers are no worse off. With allocative efficiency, the selling price is equal to the marginal cost.

The concept of efficiency in terms of improvements which, in their own judgement, benefited some people without harming others was first articulated by Vilfredo Pareto. For this reason, the term **Pareto efficiency** or **Pareto optimality** is often used synonymously with allocative efficiency but implicit in the definition of Pareto efficiency is the inclusion of technical efficiency. Pareto stressed the importance of personal judgement in defining welfare. Therefore, Pareto efficiency offers no guidance on how to make judgements on changes in the distribution of resources among individuals (*see also under* **Equity** and **Utility**).

Elasticity

Elasticity is a measure of how responsive one variable is to another. For example, price elasticity of demand measures how responsive demand (Q) is to price (P). Demand is described as elastic if the percentage or proportionate change in demand is higher than the percentage or proportionate change in price.

$$\text{Price elasticity of demand} = E = \left| \frac{\frac{dQ}{Q}}{\frac{dP}{P}} \right| \approx \left| \frac{\frac{\Delta Q}{\bar{Q}}}{\frac{\Delta P}{\bar{P}}} \right|$$

where dQ/dP is the rate of change of demand as a function of price (i.e. the inverse of the slope of the demand curve). In practice, the infinitesimally small changes dQ and dP are often approximated by the small changes ΔQ and ΔP and the corresponding points Q and P by the midpoint averages $\bar{Q}$ and $\bar{P}$.

When the percentage change in quantity demanded is less than the percentage change in price, the demand is said to be inelastic. The midpoint of a linear demand curve always has unit elasticity. Elasticity is a general concept which has been applied to various economic issues such as investment and income. In pharmacoeconomics, elasticity has been used in sensitivity analysis to test the robustness of results of cost-effectiveness studies (Einarson TR, Arikian SR, Doyle JJ (1995) Rank order stability analysis. *Medical Decision Making*. **15**: 367–72).

EM algorithm

The EM or expectation-maximization algorithm is a computational itera-tive algorithm which is particularly useful in maximum likelihood estima-tion. Although its roots date back to much earlier, the work of Dempster and colleagues popularized the method. The estimation step involves calculating the expected value of the log likelihood conditional on the observed data and the current parameter estimates. This function is then maximized to obtain updated estimates. The increased likelihood is then used in the next iteration and the whole process repeated until conver-gence is achieved (Dempster AP, Laird NM, Rubin DB (1977) Maximum-likelihood from incomplete data via the EM algorithm. *Journal of the Royal Statistical Society Series B.* **39**: 1–38. Meng XL, van Dyk D (1997) The EM algorithm – an old folk song sung to a fast new tune. *Journal of the Royal Statistical Society Series B.* **59**: 511–68).

EPACT

EPACT refers to electronic PACT, the electronically accessible information on general practitioners' prescribing in the United Kingdom (Majeed A, Evans N, Head P (1997) What can PACT tell us about prescribing in gen-eral practice? *BMJ.* **315**: 1515–19).

Equipoise

A state of uncertainty about the relative benefits and harms associated with treatments which are to be compared. Under those circumstances, a clinical trial is indicated since there are no ethical concerns about randomly assigning the treatments.

Equity

Equity and efficiency represent the two major objectives of economic policy. Equity refers to fairness. Difficulties arise in defining equity since it may, among other definitions, mean (i) giving everyone an equal share; (ii) giving everyone what they need; (iii) ensuring that everyone has access to at least a socially acceptable minimum standard of care. The term 'hori-zontal equity' is used for the principle that people in similar circumstances should be treated similarly. In contrast, the term 'vertical equity' is used for the principle that fair treatment of people in dissimilar circumstances should reflect those dissimilarities (Mooney G (1982) *Equity in health care: confronting the confusion.* Discussion Paper No. 11/82. Health Economics Research Unit, University of Aberdeen).

Equivalence studies

Equivalence studies are aimed at demonstrating that two treatments or formulations are equivalent either in efficacy or bioavailability (*see* **Bioequivalence studies**). For example, if a manufacturer plans to introduce a new formulation of an existing drug produced by another manufacturer, drug licensing authorities require evidence that it is bioequivalent to the existing product (i.e. has the same bioavailability). Otherwise, evidence of equivalent clinical effects, which is much more expensive to generate, has to be provided. For a new drug, however, as opposed to a new formulation, many manufacturers undertake equivalence studies to show that the product is as effective as an existing drug. They then justify the introduction of the new drug on the basis of greater safety or lower cost.

Estimator

An estimator is a function of observable random variables, used to estimate a parameter. The sample mean ($\bar{x}$), which is a function of sample observations, for example, can be used as an estimator of the population mean (μ). An estimator is said to be unbiased if its expected value is equal to the parameter being estimated.

European Free Trade Association (EFTA)

With the signing of the Treaty of Rome in 1957, Belgium, France, West Germany, Italy, Luxembourg and The Netherlands established the European Economic Community (EEC). Several countries, including Britain, which were part of the early negotiations, while supportive of intra-European trade, were unhappy about the establishment of the pan-European administrative structures which formation of the EEC led to. As a result, those non-EEC countries, including the Scandinavian countries, Portugal, Switzerland, Austria and Britain, formed the European Free Trade Association (EFTA) in 1960 which would abolish tariffs on mutual trade but would allow each partner to determine its own tariff on trade with non-partner countries. Soon after, the UK applied for membership of the EEC. In 1973 Britain formally joined the EEC along with Ireland and Denmark.

European Union

The European Union is an association of 12 European states working as an economic union which, in addition to forming a common market, is committed to harmonization of their general economic, legal and social policies. One of the aims of the European Union under the Treaty of

Maastricht (1993) is monetary union and hence a common currency and monetary policy. This commitment is being severely challenged in several countries of the Union. However, several countries have already adopted a common currency, the Euro.

The European Union has its roots in the formation in 1944 of the Benelux, a customs union (i.e. intra-union free trade and a common tariff on all members' trade with non-members) involving Belgium, Luxembourg and The Netherlands. This was followed by the formation of the European Coal and Steel Community (ECSC) in 1951 by the Treaty of Paris, with the objective of stimulating the recovery of heavy industries in West Germany without the latter being able to use the output to wage war again. The resulting common market (i.e. in addition to a customs union, further trade and economic integration through free mobility of factors of production and harmonization of trading standards and practices are promoted) in coal, steel and iron involved the Benelux countries, France, Italy and West Germany. The Treaty of Rome (1957) led to further European economic integration with the formation of the European Economic Community (EEC) and an atomic energy community (EURATOM). These bodies eventually merged, leading to the establishment of the European Communities (EC) in 1967 and the European Union (EU) in 1993. Current member states are the Benelux countries, Denmark, France, Germany, Greece, Ireland, Italy, Portugal, Spain and the United Kingdom.

The governance of the EU is shared between a commission, a council, a court of justice and a parliament. The Council comprises the heads of governments of the member states, usually acting through the ministers or permanent officials concerned with the relevant issues. The Council shares power with a commission comprising 17 members, appointed by the member states for four-year terms and a president appointed for two years by the Council. The Court of Justice, comprising judges appointed by member states but not removable by them to ensure that they retain independence from member governments, interprets Community law and their findings are binding on member governments. The European Government is a consultative body for both the Commission and the Council before deciding on various issues. While the Parliament may dismiss the Commission, in practice its powers are currently rather limited but likely to grow in future (Swann D (1995) *The economics of the Common Market*. 8th edn. Penguin, Harmondsworth).

Event history analysis

Event history analysis is the mathematical modelling or analysis of discrete events, such as occurrence of adverse reactions, development of epileptic fits or hospitalization, over time. In this type of analysis allowance can be made for two features which are characteristic of such data: **censoring** and time-varying explanatory variables. Application of standard statistical procedures to the analysis of such data can lead to serious bias or imprecise estimates. Event history analysis is also referred to as 'longitudinal data analysis' (Diggle PJ, Liang KY, Zeger SL (1994) *Analysis of longitudinal data.* Oxford Science Press, Oxford (for clinical applications). Allison PD (1984) *Event history analysis.* Sage Publications, Newbury (for applications in the social sciences)).

Evidence-based clinical guidelines (see also under Clinical practice guidelines)

Clinical practice guidelines are documents which are developed, usually by groups of experts, to provide advice on the best management of particular clinical conditions. Such guidelines are described as evidence-based (EBCG) if they are based on a systematic evaluation of the best available external evidence. In many areas of therapy, there is no clinical trial evidence on which to base decisions. In such cases, there is controversy about whether EBCG should provide guidance (Green L (1998) JNC VI guidelines. *Lancet.* **351**: 288).

Evidence-based health care (EBHC)

In line with the definition for **evidence-based medicine** (EBM), evidence-based health care (EBHC) can be defined as the conscientious, explicit and judicious use of current best evidence in making decisions about any aspect of health care. Using this definition, EBM can be considered to be a subset of EBHC. The latter would also include evidence-based nursing (EBN), evidence-based pharmacotherapy (EBPh), evidence-based practice (EBPr), evidence-based purchasing (EBPu), evidence-based patient choice (EBPC), evidence-based diagnosis and so on.

Note, however, that there is much controversy about the various definitions, particularly in relation to the type of evidence which is admissible, which type of evidence is best and how inclusive the evidence ought to be. The definition proposed above adopts a neutral stance in these respects. It does not take on board all the qualifiers applied by Sackett *et al.* (Sackett DL, Rosenberg WM, Gray JA *et al.* (1996) Evidence-based medicine: what it is and what it isn't. *BMJ.* **312**: 71–2) but neither does it adopt the more jaundiced approach suggested by 'When I use a word, it means exactly what I want it to mean, nothing more and nothing less'. For a discussion of best evidence, see Green G, Wennberg J, Sackett D (1997) Best evidence. *BMJ.* **315**: 1636.

Evidence-based medicine (EBM)

Evidence-based medicine has been defined as 'the conscientious, explicit and judicious use of current best evidence in making decisions about the care of individual patients' by Sackett and his colleagues who have been largely responsible for popularizing EBM as a concept (Sackett DL, Haynes RB, Guyatt GH, Tugwell P (1991) *Clinical epidemiology: a basic science for clinical medicine*. 2nd edn. Little, Brown, Boston. Sackett DL, Richardson WS, Rosenberg W, Haynes RB (1997) *Evidence-based medicine*. Churchill Livingstone, London). Those authors also stress that the practice of EBM means integrating individual clinical expertise with the best available external evidence from systematic search. However, the term EBM is now used much more generally to mean the systematic, explicit and judicious use of best evidence in patient care (*see also* **Evidence-based pharmacotherapy** and **Evidence-based purchasing**).

Evidence-based medicine resource list

This is an Internet site maintained by the library at the University of Hertfordshire. It carries a range of useful references and links to various other sites (*see* http://www.herts.ac.uk/lrc/subjects/health/ebm.htm).

Evidence-based pharmacotherapy (EBPh)

Evidence-based pharmacotherapy is the systematic, explicit and judicious use of best evidence in making decisions about drug treatment for patients, at both the individual and population (policy) levels. When defining the pharmacotherapeutic profile of a drug, in addition to risk-benefit considerations, the economic aspects are evaluated so that the most cost-effective treatments can be adopted. A decision analytic framework which incorporates patients' preferences, comorbidities and risk factors should be adopted when applying evidence-based pharmacotherapy at the level of the individual patient.

Evidence-based purchasing

Evidence-based purchasing refers to the purchasing of services (e.g. stroke services) on the basis of a rigorous examination of the scientific evidence. In particular, cost-effectiveness issues need to be carefully assessed when purchasing services on behalf of the community. *Evidence-based Purchasing* is also the title of a bimonthly digest of evidence about effective care published by the Research Directorate of the UK South and West Regional Health Authority (http://www.epi.bris.ac.uk/rd/publica/ebpurch).

Excess risk

In a comparative study of risks associated with exposure to two therapies or environments, the difference in risk can be expressed in absolute or relative terms (*see* **Risk difference**, **Relative risk** and **Risk ratio**). The ratio of the risk associated with one exposure divided by the risk associated with the other is the relative risk. Suppose that the risk of developing diarrhoea after receiving a course of antibiotic A is 5 in 100 and 2 in 100 for antibiotic B, then the relative risk of developing this side-effect when receiving A instead of B is 2.5 (i.e. 0.05/0.02). The excess risk is the difference in risk expressed as a percentage or 150% in this case (i.e. $100 \times (5-2)/2$). A common mistake in the literature is to interpret a risk ratio or relative risk of 2.5 as a 250% or two and a half-fold increase in risk (Lam TH (1997) Relative risks are inflated in published literature. *BMJ*. **315**: 880).

Explanatory trial analysis (*see under* Intention to treat analysis)

Exponential survival model

The exponential survival model is characterized by the following survival function, where T is a random variable representing failure time:

$$S(t) = P(T \leqslant t) = \exp(-\lambda t)$$

The corresponding probability density function is given by $f(y) = \lambda \exp(-\lambda t)$. The mean μ of the exponential distribution is given by $1/\lambda$ and its variance σ^2 by $1/\lambda^2$. The shape of the survival curve is of the type shown in Figure 8.

Expressed preference method (*see under* Willingness to pay)

External validity

External validity refers to how applicable the results of a study are to the target population. For example, a frequently expressed concern is whether conclusions drawn from the results of clinical trials using patients adhering to strict inclusion criteria are applicable to the population of patients visiting primary care physicians. In other words, critics question the external validity or **generalizability** of such clinical trial data to the average primary care patient.

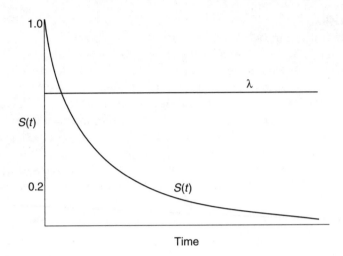

Figure 8 Exponential survival model

Externality

Allocative efficiency occurs when the marginal benefits equal the marginal costs. In a number of instances, the marginal private cost (that which the consumer pays) does not fully reflect the marginal cost to society. A classic example arises when manufacturing of a particular product causes pollution. The additional cost of cleaning up the environment is not usually reflected in the market price of the product and can hence be viewed as the subsidy provided by society to the consumer of the product. Such costs are referred to as external costs or externalities. In the presence of a negative externality (E), a quantity (Q1) which is more than the optimum quantity (Q0) of the product is produced and the resources are not allocated efficiently (Figure 9). Externalities can be positive too. For example, by vaccinating a child, not only is the child better protected from the potential invading micro-organism but society as a whole benefits from lower transmission rates of the infection through the development of herd immunity. It has also been argued that human beings generally do not like to see others suffer from untreated illness and that they care for the welfare of others. Therefore, there is associated with health care a positive caring externality (Culyer AJ (1980) *The political economy of social policy*. Martin Robertson, Oxford).

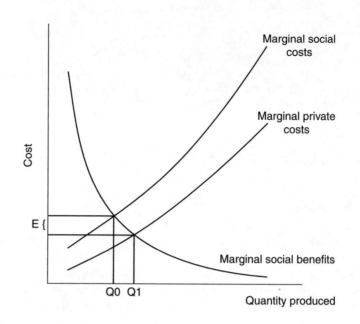

Figure 9 Concept of externality

Factor cost (*see under* **Gross domestic product**)

Fail-safe number

For a variety of reasons, notably the preference of authors to submit studies with positive results rather than negative results for publication, studies in the former group are more likely to be published. Therefore estimates of effect based on the results of studies in the public domain may be biased. Therefore when undertaking meta-analyses, a critical assessment of the potential threats to the validity of the estimates of effect is necessary. Rosenthal suggested calculating the number of studies needed to nullify any effect observed (Rosenthal R (1979) The 'file drawer problem' and tolerance of null results. *Psychological Bulletin.* **86**: 638–41) and Cooper suggested calling this number the 'fail-safe sample size' (Cooper H (1979) Statistically combining independent studies: a meta-analysis of sex differences in conformity research. *Journal of Personality and Social Psychology.* **37**: 131–46). This number, which is now generally referred to as the fail-safe number, is calculated as follows:

Suppose that there are k published studies and the significance level for these studies are $p_1, p_2, p_3, \ldots, p_k$. Postulate the null hypothesis that the mean effect is zero and that each p_i is uniformly distributed on [0, 1]. Let Z_i be the standard normal variate associated with each p_i. Z_i is then given by $Z_i = \Phi^{-1}(1 - p_i)$ where Φ is the standard normal cumulative distribution function. Let $S_k = Z_1 + Z_2 + \ldots + Z_n$ and z_α be the critical value for a one-sided test at a significance level of α for a normally distributed mean effect. The fail-safe N is then calculated by solving the following equation.

$$\frac{S_k}{\sqrt{(k+n)}} = z_\alpha$$

Fallacy of composition

The fallacy of composition is the error made by wrongly generalizing to groups the results which apply to individuals. In economic theory, two phenomena, the paradox of thrift and the tragedy of the commons, are examples of fallacy of composition. The former relates to the observation that if one person saves a higher proportion of his wages to purchase a specific item, he will acquire that item sooner than otherwise. On the other hand, if everyone were to save more, for the economy as a whole, the absolute total amount saved could actually be less since output and hence employment would drop. As a result, there is less money to be saved. The tragedy of the commons can be illustrated by the fact that if farmers were allowed to graze their sheep on public land for free and one farmer were to increase his herd, then he would be better off. On the other hand, if every farmer were to do the same, overgrazing may follow and everybody would be worse off.

False-negative ratio

The false-negative ratio in diagnostic testing is the proportion of negative tests $(-T)$ in all patients with disease (D).

False-negative ratio $= p(-T|D)$

False-positive ratio

The false-positive ratio in diagnostic testing is the proportion of positive tests $(+T)$ in patients without disease.

False-positive ratio $= p(+T|\bar{D})$

Field trial

Unlike a clinical trial which deals with patients, a field trial is one which deals with individuals who have yet to develop the disease. Such trials usually involve large numbers of subjects going about their usual daily activities. Therefore, the investigators usually visit their subjects in the field (workplace, school or home). Field studies are commonly used for studying the efficacy of vaccines (Rothman KJ, Greenland S (1998) *Modern epidemiology*. 2nd edn. Lippincott-Raven, Philadelphia).

File drawer problem

The term 'file drawer problem' was first coined by Rosenthal to describe the publication bias which results from authors and editors favouring the publication of studies with positive results (Rosenthal R (1979) The 'file drawer problem' and tolerance of null results. *Psychological Bulletin.* **86**: 638–41). As a result, estimates of the efficacy of drugs based solely on data available in the public domain are often over-optimistic. To minimize such a problem, reviewers are advised to seek access to unpublished studies from likely investigators and product manufacturers. However, the latter are often reluctant to make such information available.

Fiscal policy

Fiscal policy is the policy adopted by a government with respect to taxes and government spending to influence its economic targets.

Five-year survival rate (*see under* Case fatality rate)

Fixed costs

Fixed costs are those which remain constant when the level of output changes. For example, in the manufacture of tablets, the cost of the tabletting machine is a fixed cost as it is required whether the level of output is high or low as long as the machine's capacity is not exceeded.

Floor effect (*see under* Ceiling effect)

Focus groups

Focus groups are one of the qualitative research methods based on group interviews. With this approach, a moderator poses open-ended questions to a group of participants drawn from a target population of interest. The method is widely used in marketing research, for example, to tap into what a group of primary care physicians might think about the profile of a new drug or how health education messages are likely to be perceived.

Unlike one-to-one interviews, in focus groups, group dynamics can be capitalized on to clarify complex issues and unravel interaction between different factors. In the real world, individuals' perceptions are often modified and perhaps even shaped by those of their peers. Focus groups may help to explore the extent to which this is likely.

In modern practice, focus groups are often conducted by professional moderators while those commissioning or undertaking the research observe, with the participants' permission, through video link-ups. The video tapes can be subject to subsequent further analysis. Additional questions may be conveyed by the observers to the moderators at inter-missions. Indeed, the participants themselves are encouraged to generate new questions for group exploration. Throughout the sessions, an informal atmosphere is encouraged through proper seating arrangements and with exchange of personal experiences, jokes and anecdotes. Group norms about highly sensitive issues such as sexual behaviour and cultural values can then be explored. Subjects who cannot read or write can participate and with skilful moderation, the more reticent can contribute fully to the discussions (Morgan D (1988) *Focus groups as qualitative research*. Sage, London. Kreugerk RA (1988) *Focus groups: a practical guide for applied research*. Sage, London).

Follow-up study (see *also* under Cohort study)
A prospective study in which subjects are recruited and followed forward in time.

Food and Drug Administration (FDA)
The FDA of the United States is the country's food and drug regulatory authority. It sets standards which manufacturers are advised to adopt or which they must meet in order to obtain marketing authorization (*see* website www.fda.gov).

(The) Fundamental economic problem (see Economic problem)

Fundholding
This refers to the scheme initiated by the UK Department of Health whereby primary care physicians (general practitioners or GPs) were able to volunteer to hold a budget with which to buy services for their patients. With a budget, they could determine allocation for the different types of services on offer and savings made in one area (e.g. expenditure on drugs) could be used elsewhere (e.g. services of a diabetes adviser or additional nurse). Savings could not be used for personal gain except indirectly such as through capital investments to improve their premises.

By the end of 1996, over 50% of GPs were fundholders in some capacity. A recent report by the UK Audit Commission suggests that only in some 10% of GP fundholding practices had benefits been gained by patients. Fundholding is being reorganized into consortia or **primary care groups** for given geographical areas to care for patient groups of about 100 000 in size (DoH (1997) *The new NHS*. Cmd 3807. HMSO, London).

Funnel plot

This is a graphical method often used for identifying possible publication bias when undertaking a systematic overview. The effect measures are plotted against the corresponding sample sizes as exemplified in Figure 10. In the absence of publication bias, the points should be distributed in a roughly symmetric manner to outline the shape of an inverted funnel. Withholding publication of studies with small or no significant effects leads to truncation of the left side of the inverted funnel. Estimates of effect obtained by undertaking a meta-analysis of published studies will there-fore tend to be too high. However, an asymmetric funnel plot does not necessarily indicate publication bias. It may be due to true heterogeneity or real differences in the effects between trials (Egger M, Smith GD, Schneider M, Minder C (1997) Bias in meta-analysis detected by a simple graphical test. *BMJ*. **315**: 629–34. Stuck AE, Rubenstein LZ, Wieland D (1998) Asymmetry detected in funnel plot was probably due to true heterogeneity. *BMJ*. **316**: 469).

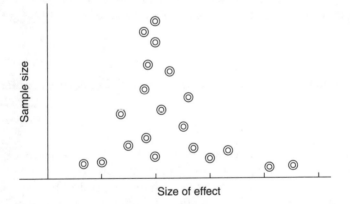

Figure 10 Funnel plot

Game theory

Game theory, first developed by **von Neumann** (1903–57), is the study of strategic decision making by more than one person. A classic application of game theory is in the study of oligopolies or markets in which there are a few firms, each of which has to consider the response of others before acting. In such a market, before a firm raises or drops its prices, it has to consider whether the others will follow or take no action. Using game theory, it can be shown that in such a market, the oligopolists are likely to maintain price stability (von Neumann J, Morgenstern O (1944) *The theory of games and economic behaviour*. John Wiley, New York. Gibbons R (1992) *A primer in game theory*. Harvester Wheatsheaf, Hertfordshire).

GCP (see **Good clinical practice**)

GDP deflator

The gross domestic product (GDP) deflator is a number which shows the GDP in constant prices. It is derived by dividing the GDP in current prices by the GDP in constant prices. When presenting the GDP deflator for a number of years in the form of a series, scaling is used. A given year is used as the reference year and given a value of 100. For example, in the 1994 US Economic Report to the President, the GDP deflator for 1987 was assigned a value of 100. The deflators for 1985, 1986, 1987, 1988, 1989 and 1990 were given as 94.4, 96.6, 100, 103.9, 108.5 and 113.3 respectively. Therefore, given the deflator for a given year and the GDP for that year, the GDP can be expressed in 1987 dollars.

General Household Survey

The General Household Survey (GHS) is an annual survey undertaken by the UK Office for National Statistics (ONS) to provide data on health, population characteristics, education and economic activity. The need for the GHS is being reviewed by the ONS.

Generalizability (see **External validity**)

Generalizability theory

Classic test theory assumes that an observed test score is made up of two components, a true score and an error term. The ratio of the true variance to the composite (true + error) variance is the reliability coefficient.

Generalizability theory proposes that whenever measurements are taken, there are many sources of variance (referred to as facets) contributing error to the estimates being made. An important objective of any estimation is therefore the identification and measurement of those variance components through appropriate factorial studies. Such studies are referred to as generalizability or G studies in the literature relating to development of measurement scales. Within the framework of generalizability theory, studies are also undertaken to evaluate how decision rules, such as pooling of different raters' scores, influence the reliability of the measurements. Such studies are called decision or D studies (Cronbach LJ, Gleser GC, Nanda H, Rajaratnam N (1972) *The dependability of behavioral measurement: theory of generalizability for scores.* John Wiley, New York).

Generalized linear model

The generalized linear model is a statistical model for analysing the pattern of association and interactions between variables which takes the form:

$$g(y) = \alpha + \beta_1 x_1 + \dots \beta_k x_k$$

Where $g(y)$ is a function of the dependent variable η, the beta values are the coefficients for the k predictor (x) variables. All generalized linear models include three components: (i) the random component which identifies the response variable; (ii) a systematic component which specifies the explanatory or predictor variables; (iii) a link which describes the functional relationship between the systematic component and the expected values of the random component.

Generalized linear models include ordinary regression analysis and analysis of variance as well as more complex models such as logistic regression models and log linear models.

Generic substitution

When drugs lose their patent, manufacturers other than the innovator company can supply alternative bioequivalent products (generic equivalents). To reduce drug costs, health care providers and hospitals may permit the supply of such products when prescribers request the innovator's branded product (generic substitution). In the UK, under the National Health Service, generic substitution is not allowed in general practice with the emphasis being placed on generic prescribing instead. When a prescriber orders a drug generically, then the pharmacist can supply any generic equivalent. In the hospital service, generic substitution is common but needs to be agreed on by the appropriate drug and therapeutic committees.

Geometric mean

The geometric mean is the antilogarithm of $\overline{\log x}$ where

$$\overline{\log x} = \frac{1}{n} \sum_{i=1}^{n} \log x_i$$

Any base can be used provided the same base is used for both the log and antilog steps. The geometric mean is often used in summarizing pharmacokinetic data such as the ratio of area under the blood concentration–time curves for the products being compared because of their non-normal distribution.

Geometric series

A geometric series is a sequence of numbers in which consecutive terms differ from each other by a constant ratio r whose modulus is smaller than one. Such a series of n terms can be written as $a, ar^2, ar^2, ar^3 \ldots, ar^{n-1}$ where $|r| < 1$ and a is the first term. The sum S_n of the n terms is given by:

$$S_n = \frac{a(r^n - 1)}{r-1} \text{ and when } n \text{ tends to infinity by } S_\infty = \frac{a}{1-r}$$

Gini coefficient

The Gini coefficient is an index which quantifies the degree of inequality in an economy. Its value ranges from 0 to 1. With perfect equality of income, the Gini coefficient takes a value of 0. A value of 1 indicates that all the income accrues to a single individual (*see under* **Lorenz curve** for a description of how it is calculated).

Global measures

In the assessment of perception, a global measure is one where the person makes a single assessment about the overall value of an intervention on his or her own status. Two types of global measures are often used in health-related quality of life assessments: (i) preference measures by which the subjects express a judgement about how much they would be prepared to sacrifice in order to achieve perfect health; (ii) rating scales by which patients rate their health status using categorical descriptive labels or analogue (continuous) scales. All rating scales are usually anchored so that the two ends of the scales refer to perfect health and as good as dead. States of health worse than death may be assigned negative values, particularly in community-derived scales.

In preference measurements, what is being traded for perfect health can be years of life, risk of death or money. The method is then referred to as time trade-off, standard gamble or willingness to pay respectively. Global values using both preference measures and rating scales can be transformed to a utility scale ranging from 0 to 1. These utilities can then be used for quality-adjusting life-years to yield QALYs, a basic unit in cost utility analyses.

Gold standard

The term 'gold standard' in measurement scale development or pharmaco-economic evaluation refers to the comparator which is generally regarded to be the best available. For example, in the survey of health status, the SF-36 form is often regarded as the gold standard. Therefore when developing or proposing a new form, it is expected that any validation would include the concurrent use of SF-36.

Good clinical practice

Good clinical practice for the conduct of a clinical trial defines what needs to be done before, during and after completion of the trial to ensure full accountability. The steps required for GCP are defined in a guideline issued by the International Conference on Harmonization (ICH) of technical requirements for registration of pharmaceuticals for human use. While the health ministries of different countries will have their own criteria, the ICH guideline summarizes the consensus views of regulatory authorities in the USA, the European Community and Japan after wide-ranging consultation with interested parties such as the pharmaceutical industry. Issues such as informed consent, ethics committee approval, randomization list, subject enrolment log and reporting of adverse drug reactions are highlighted (*see* Document E6 obtainable from the ICH Secretariat, Geneva, Switzerland).

GP fundholding (see Fundholding)

Gross domestic product (GDP)

The GDP of a country is the value of all its final output of goods and services produced within the country during the relevant period, usually a year. The final output is used to avoid double counting of primary or intermediate materials which are then converted into other goods. The GDP can be contrasted with the **gross national product** (GNP) which measures the final output of goods and services by factors of production owned by its people, irrespective of where the production takes place. The difference between the GNP and the GDP of a country therefore gives an estimate of the net national income from abroad. Both GNP and GDP can be expressed inclusive of taxes at time of sale (market prices) or excluding such taxes but including subsidies paid to the producer (factor cost).

Another related term is the net national product (NNP) which is the gross national income net of capital stock (factories and machinery) depreciation.

Gross domestic product deflator (see GDP deflator)

Gross national product (GNP) (see *under* Gross domestic product)

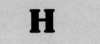

H

Hawthorne effect

This is the term (named after a study of industrial efficiency at the Hawthorne plant in Chicago) used to describe the effect which is induced by the study itself because subjects react abnormally when they know they are being observed.

Hazard function

The hazard function, a term used in survival analysis, is a measure of the potential to failure as a function of age. Let T be the random variable representing time to failure or death. The hazard function $\lambda(t)$ can then be written as:

$$\lambda(t) = \lim_{\Delta t \to 0} \frac{P(t \leqslant T < t + \Delta t | t \leqslant T)}{\Delta t}$$

The product $\lambda(t)dt$ is the probability of failure in the infinitesimally small interval $t, t + dt$ given survival at time t. The hazard function can also be written as:

$$\lambda(t) = f(t|t) = \frac{f(t)}{S(t)}$$

where $f(t)$ is the probability density function and $S(t) = 1 - f(t) = P(T > t)$ is the survival function. $f(t)$ is also called the unconditional failure rate, in contrast to the hazard function which is also referred to as the conditional failure rate. The reason for this can be seen by comparing the definition of $f(t)$ with the hazard function.

$$f(t) = \frac{dF(t)}{dt} = \lim_{\Delta t \to 0} \frac{P(t \leqslant T \leqslant t + \Delta t)}{\Delta t}$$

$f(t)$, $S(t)$ and $\lambda(t)$ are approximated as follows:

$f(t) = \dfrac{n_1}{(N)(\Delta t)}$ where n_1 is the number of deaths or failures in the interval beginning at time t

$S(t) = \dfrac{n_2}{N}$ where n_2 is the number of patients surviving longer than t

$\lambda(t) = \dfrac{n_1}{(n_3)(\Delta t)}$ where n_3 is the number of patients surviving at time t.

Health action zones

Health action zones are a new initiative proposed in the UK government's 1998 White Paper *The New NHS* to bring together organizations with an interest in health care to develop and implement locally approved strategies for improving the local delivery of health.

Health authorities

Health authorities are bodies within the UK National Health Service, set up to manage health care delivery for a specific geographical area. They allocate health care funds and hold those receiving such funds to account.

Health maintenance organization (see under Managed care)

Health-related quality of life (see Quality of life)

Health technology assessment reports

These are commissioned reports funded by the UK Department of Health under its NHS Health Technology Assessment Programme and co-ordinated by the National Co-ordinating Centre for Health Technology Assessment (http://www.soton.ac.uk/~wi/hta/htapubs.html).

Healthy cohort bias (see Bias and Healthy user bias)

Healthy user bias

This is the bias which can be introduced in observational studies when one of the groups being compared consists of healthier subjects than the other(s). For example, in a number of reported observational studies of hormone replacement therapy (HRT), the subjects in the HRT group appeared to have been healthier than the control group thereby possibly leading to erroneous protective effects being reported. Such a bias could be introduced by doctors, for example only prescribing HRT to healthy patients because of perceived contraindications to HRT such as the presence of cardiovascular disease (Grodstein F, Stampfer MJ, Colditz GA *et al.* (1997) Postmenopausal therapy and mortality. *New England Journal of Medicine.* **336**: 1769–75).

Healthy year equivalent (HYE)

Treatment may increase survival without necessarily improving the quality of life. Indeed, in certain instances, such as treatment with some chemotherapeutic regimens and surgical interventions in early prostatic cancer, treatment may in fact increase morbidity. How to decide on the best treatment is therefore difficult and there is a need to take account of patients' preferences or utilities. The HYE associated with an intervention is the gain in life-years adjusted to take account of patients' preferences measured using a two-stage lottery approach (Mehrez A, Gafni A (1989) Quality-adjusted life years, utility theory and healthy years equivalent. *Medical Decision Making.* **9**: 141–9). While the HYE overcomes the need for assuming utility functions of the same form for all individuals and is consistent with the efficiency criterion of economic theory, it is not yet widely accepted. To date, the QALY is the favoured outcome measure of gain in cost utility analyses (Culyer AJ, Wagstaff A (1993) QALYs and HYEs. *Journal of Health Economics.* **11**: 311–23).

HEAPACT

HEAPACT is an electronic link between UK health authorities and the Prescription Pricing Authority which allows the former to download computerized data about the prescribing of general practices in their areas. With HEAPACT, health authorities can obtain information about the prescribing of specific drugs in sufficient detail to, for example, identify how new drugs are being taken up by various practices (Majeed A, Evans N, Head P (1997) What can PACT tell us about prescribing in general practice? *BMJ.* **315**: 1515–19).

Helsinki Declaration

The Helsinki Declaration is a set of recommendations guiding physicians in biomedical research involving human subjects adopted by the 18th World Medical Assembly in Helsinki, 1964, and amended by the 29th World Medical Assembly in Tokyo, 1975, the 35th World Medical Assembly in Venice, 1983, and the 41st World Medical Assembly in Hong Kong, 1989, and is reproduced below.

Introduction

It is the mission of the physician to safeguard the health of the people. His or her knowledge and conscience are dedicated to the fulfilment of this mission. The Declaration of Geneva of the World Medical Association binds the physician with the words, 'The health of my patient will be my first consideration,' and the International Code of Medical Ethics declares that, 'A physician shall act only in the patient's interest when providing medical care which might have the effect of weakening the physical and mental condition of the patient.'

The purpose of biomedical research involving human subjects must be to improve diagnostic, therapeutic and prophylactic procedures and the understanding of the aetiology and pathogenesis of disease. In current medical practice most diagnostic, therapeutic or prophylactic procedures involve hazards. This applies especially to biomedical research. Medical progress is based on research which ultimately must rest in part on experimentation involving human subjects. In the field of biomedical research a fundamental distinction must be recognized between medical research in which the aim is essentially diagnostic or therapeutic for a patient, and medical research, the essential object of which is purely scientific and without implying direct diagnostic or therapeutic value to the person subjected to the research. Special caution must be exercised in the conduct of research which may affect the environment, and the welfare of animals used for research must be respected. Because it is essential that the results of laboratory experiments be applied to human beings to further scientific knowledge and to help suffering humanity, the World Medical Association has prepared the following recommendations as a guide to every physician in biomedical research involving human subjects. They should be kept under review in the future. It must be stressed that the standards as drafted are only a guide to physicians all over the world. Physicians are not relieved from criminal, civil and ethical responsibilities under the law of their own countries.

I Basic principles

1 Biomedical research involving human subjects must conform to generally accepted scientific principles and should be based on adequately

performed laboratory and animal experimentation and on a thorough knowledge of the scientific literature.

2 The design and performance of each experimental procedure involving human subjects should be clearly formulated in an experimental protocol which should be transmitted for consideration, comment and guidance to a specially appointed committee independent of the investigator and the sponsor provided that this independent committee is in conformity with the laws and regulations of the country in which the research experiment is performed.

3 Biomedical research involving human subjects should be conducted only by scientifically qualified persons and under the supervision of a clinically competent medical person. The responsibility for the human subject must always rest with a medically qualified person and never rest on the subject of the research, even though the subject has given his or her consent.

4 Biomedical research involving human subjects cannot legitimately be carried out unless the importance of the objective is in proportion to the inherent risk to the subject.

5 Every biomedical research project involving human subjects should be preceded by careful assessment of predictable risks in comparison with foreseeable benefits to the subject or to others. Concern for the interests of the subject must always prevail over the interests of science and society.

6 The right of the research subject to safeguard his or her integrity must always be respected. Every precaution should be taken to respect the privacy of the subject and to minimize the impact of the study on the subject's physical and mental integrity and on the personality of the subject.

7 Physicians should abstain from engaging in research projects involving human subjects unless they are satisfied that the hazards involved are believed to be predictable. Physicians should cease any investigation if the hazards are found to outweigh the potential benefits.

8 In publication of the results of his or her research, the physician is obliged to preserve the accuracy of the results. Reports of experimentation not in accordance with the principles laid down in this Declaration should not be accepted for publication.

9 In any research on human beings, each potential subject must be adequately informed of the aims, methods, anticipated benefits and potential hazards of the study and the discomfort it may entail. He or she should be informed that he or she is at liberty to abstain from participation in the study and that he or she is free to withdraw his or her consent to participation at any time. The physician should then obtain the subject's freely given informed consent, preferably in writing.

10 When obtaining informed consent for the research project the physician should be particularly cautious if the subject is in a dependent relationship to him or her or may consent under duress. In that case the informed consent should be obtained by a physician who is not engaged in the investigation and who is completely independent of this official relationship.

11 In case of legal incompetence, informed consent should be obtained from the legal guardian in accordance with national legislation. Where physical or mental incapacity makes it impossible to obtain informed consent, or when the subject is a minor, permission from the responsible relative replaces that of the subject in accordance with national legislation. Whenever the minor child is in fact able to give a consent, the minor's consent must be obtained in addition to the consent of the minor's legal guardian.

12 The research protocol should always contain a statement of the ethical considerations involved and should indicate that the principles enunciated in the present Declaration are complied with.

II Medical research combined with professional care (clinical research)
1 In the treatment of the sick person, the physician must be free to use a new diagnostic and therapeutic measure, if in his or her judgement it offers hope of saving life, re-establishing health or alleviating suffering.

2 The potential benefits, hazards and discomfort of a new method should be weighed against the advantages of the best current diagnostic and therapeutic methods.

3 In any medical study, every patient – including those of a control group, if any – should be assured of the best proven diagnostic and therapeutic method.

4 The refusal of the patient to participate in a study must never interfere with the physician–patient relationship.

5 If the physician considers it essential not to obtain informed consent, the specific reasons for this proposal should be stated in the experimental protocol for transmission to the independent committee (I, 2).

6 The physician can combine medical research with professional care, the objective being the acquisition of new medical knowledge, only to the extent that medical research is justified by its potential diagnostic or therapeutic value for the patient.

III Non-therapeutic biomedical research involving human subjects (non-clinical biomedical research)
1 In the purely scientific application of medical research carried out on a human being, it is the duty of the physician to remain the protector of the life and health of that person on whom biomedical research is being carried out.

2 The subjects should be volunteers – either healthy persons or patients for whom the experimental design is not related to the patient's illness.

3 The investigator or the investigating team should discontinue the research if in his/her or their judgement it may, if continued, be harmful to the individual.

4 In research on man, the interests of science and society should never take precedence over considerations related to the well-being of the subject.

Heterogeneity
In the literature on **evidence-based medicine**, heterogeneity refers to non-homogeneous treatment effects (statistical heterogeneity) or patient groups (clinical heterogeneity) across trials. The latter and differences in treatment protocols will contribute to statistical heterogeneity (Thompson SG (1995) Why sources of heterogeneity in meta-analysis should be investigated. In: Chalmers I, Altman DG (eds) *Systematic reviews*. BMJ Publishing Group, London).

HMO (see **Health maintenance organizations**)

Human capital method
In economics, human capital is defined generally as the level of skills and knowledge which the workforce has as a result of education and training.

It is used in many areas of economics such as modelling of economic growth. In the health economics literature, the human capital method is used for estimating the loss in productivity (indirect cost) due to illness. In its simplest form, consider a previously fully healthy individual who succumbs to disease. The illness takes its course and the patient recovers to be fully fit again. The time off work can hence be ascertained and a value placed on that based on market earnings. The modelling clearly needs to be much more complex if disease incapacity is preceded by a period of ill health which reduces productivity or recovery is accompanied by residual morbidity. The human capital approach is now rarely used because it discriminates against people not earning a wage and because it is not rooted in the theoretical foundations of cost benefit analysis where benefits are defined as the willingness to pay for those benefits (Becker GS (1964) *Human capital*. University of Chicago Press, Chicago. Berger MC, Blomquist GC, Kenkel G, Tolley GS (1989) Valuing changes in health risks: a comparison of alternative measures. *Southern Economic Journal*. **53**: 967–84).

Human development index

The human development index (HDI) is a measure of living standards proposed by the United Nations Development Program in 1990 to account for the contribution of factors other than the gross domestic product (GDP) to human well-being. In addition to GDP at purchasing power parity on a sliding scale, the index includes life expectancy at birth, income, adult literacy and enrolment in primary, secondary and tertiary education. In the 1994 world rankings, Canada took pole position based on HDI, while it was only eighth when ranked on per capita GDP. France took the second and 15th positions on the two corresponding rankings. In contrast, Singapore and Hong Kong had higher per capita GDP than HDI rankings (*Economist* (1997) **343**: 138).

Hypothesis testing

Often we need to ask questions such as whether, after a given treatment, the weight of those treated has changed relative to those receiving a placebo. To answer such questions objectively, in classic statistics, one starts off with a null hypothesis (H_0). This is a statistical hypothesis that one postulates and against which we would test the observed data. It contains a statement about what one believes about the value of one or more population parameters or about the probabilistic mechanism which has generated the observations. For example, we may wish to compare the effects of a new antihypertensive agent against an established one. To test for this we postulate that the two drugs are of equal efficacy. This forms our null hypothesis which can be written symbolically as:

$$H_0: \mu_1 = \mu_2 \quad \text{or} \quad H_0: \mu_1 - \mu_2 = 0$$

In a hypothesis test we also have to specify an alternative hypothesis (H_1) which we would accept if our null hypothesis is rejected. The simple alternative for the above example is that the two drugs do not produce similar average effects. This can be written as:

$$H_1: \mu_1 \neq \mu_2 \quad \text{or} \quad H_1: \mu_1 - \mu_2 \neq 0$$

In a hypothesis test, we also have to define the significance level of the test. This is the probability at which we would reject the null hypothesis. For example, we may postulate that the effects of the two drugs are normally distributed. Under this assumption, we may say that if the observed difference in mean effects of the two drugs is so extreme (under our null hypothesis of equipotency) that they would only occur with a probability of 0.05 or lower, then we would reject the null hypothesis and accept the alternative hypothesis. This 0.05 value is what we call the significance level of our test (see Li Wan Po A (1998) *Statistics for pharmacists*. Blackwell Science, Oxford).

ICD (see *International Classification of Diseases*)

ICD-9-CM

ICD-9-CM is a classification of medical procedures based on the ninth revision of the *International Classification of Diseases* published by the World Health Organization. The hierarchical classification uses up to four digits to classify a particular procedure. For example, all operations on the cardiovascular system are coded with a first digit 3. Operations on the valves and septa of the heart are given a code of 35. Closed heart valvotomy, which is in the next hierarchical level, is given the code 35.0 and closed heart valvotomy involving the mitral valve 35.02 (ICD-9-CM. International classification of diseases (9th revision) (1994) *Clinical modification*. 4th edition. US Dept of Health and Human Services, Washington DC).

ICH

The International Conferences on Harmonization (ICH) are a series of conferences organized by the drug regulatory agencies of the USA, the European Community and Japan to develop consensus positions about various technical requirements for registration of pharmaceuticals for human use. Examples of issues considered include genotoxicity tests for pharmaceuticals, structure and content of clinical study reports and carcinogenicity studies of pharmaceuticals. Expert working parties are set up to draft guidelines (grey report, stage 2 of the ICH process) which are issued to various interested parties, notably the pharmaceutical industry, for comment. The comments are considered and ICH harmonized tripartite guidelines agreed on at steering committee meetings held in one of the three regions. Those guidelines (yellow reports, stage 4 of the ICH process) are issued with the recommendation that they be adopted by the three regulatory parties. Further information may be obtained from the secretariat: IFPMA, 30 Rue de St Jean, PO Box 9, 1211 Geneva 18, Switzerland. Fax +41-223458275.

Impact lag

The impact lag refers to the time it takes for the effects of a policy change to be felt. In monetary policy the impact lag may be close to a year and in fiscal policy, wide variability in impact lag has been observed (*see* **Implementation lag** and **Recognition lag**).

Implementation lag

The implementation lag refers to the time delay between identification of the need to institute a policy change and its actual implementation. In health care, for example, the need to change treatment protocol based on high-quality clinical trial evidence (e.g. use of thrombolysis in the management of post-myocardial patients) may be followed by guideline development and then adoption by prescribers, a sequence which is associated with well-known and reported implementation lags (European Secondary Prevention Study Group (1996) Translation of clinical trials into practice: a European population-based study of the use of thrombolysis for acute myocardial infarction. *Lancet.* **347**: 1203–7). (*See also* **Impact lag** and **Recognition lag**).

Inception cohort

In studies designed to investigate prognosis, a group of patients at a common point in the course of the disease under investigation is recruited. Clearly, the earlier the recruitment in the course of the disease, the easier it is to be comprehensive about the prognostic factors. A group of patients recruited as soon as the disease becomes clinically identifiable is referred to as an inception cohort.

Incidence

The incidence of an event (e.g. disease or adverse reaction) refers to the frequency of new cases in the population at risk during a specified time interval. The prevalence, on the other hand, refers to the frequency of all current cases in the population at risk at a specific time (point prevalence) or time interval (period prevalence). Mathematically, the prevalence (P) is approximately equal to the incidence (I) multiplied by the duration (T) of the disease ($P = I \times T$). Figure 11 illustrates which cases are included when calculating incidence and prevalence.

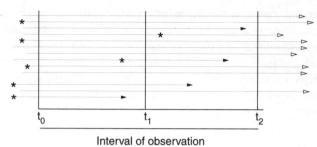

Interval of observation

★ = onset of chronic disease
► = death
At t_1 prevalence = $\frac{5}{12}$
At t_2 prevalence = $\frac{4}{9}$

Over study period only two incident cases are observed
and included in calculation of incidence rate.

Figure 11 Identification of cases included in the calculation of incidence and prevalence

Incidence study (see also under Cohort study)

A study in which subjects are recruited and followed forward in time so
that the rate at which particular events of interest occur can be recorded to
enable calculation of incidence.

Incremental cost

The incremental cost is the difference between the cost of an intervention
and the cost of the programme to which it is compared. More generally, the
term 'incremental cost' is used synonymously with the term 'marginal
cost' which is the cost of producing the last unit of product, as illustrated
in Table 2 below.

Table 2 The relationship between average and marginal costs

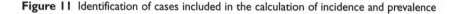

Output	Average cost	Total cost	Marginal cost
1	10	10	10
2	8	16	6
3	7	21	5
4	6.25	25	4
5	5.8	29	4
6	5.8	34.8	5.8
7	6	42	7.2

Note that the marginal cost is calculated by subtracting from the last total cost, the previous total.

In **incremental cost-effectiveness analysis**, estimated incremental costs are divided by the estimated incremental number of effectiveness units to give an incremental **cost-effectiveness ratio** (CER). In a multitreatment comparison, the incremental CER should be calculated relative to the next most effective mutually exclusive alternative (*see* **Dominance**) (Weinstein MC, Zeckhauser R (1973) Clinical ratios and efficient allocation. *Journal of Public Economics.* **2**: 147–57).

IND

An IND is an investigational new drug in relation to drug licence applications to the US Food and Drug Administration.

Index date

In a case-control study, subjects are recruited to identify association between an adverse event (e.g. pulmonary hypertension) and exposure to a putative risk factor (e.g. anorectic agents). Cases (e.g. patients with pulmonary hypertension) identified and matched controls are then interviewed to assess exposure to the risk factor (e.g. anorectic drugs) and presence of confounding factors (e.g. high body mass index, drug abuse or smoking). The index date is the date from which the cases and controls recruited are asked to recall their exposure history to the various risk factors (e.g. date from which they first perceived a symptom such as dyspnoea in assessing pulmonary hypertension).

Indifference curve

We are often put in a position of having to choose relative amounts of different goods which we would like to have at least some of (e.g. food and medicine or extent and quality of life; my students like to consider the trade-off between beer and food). An indifference curve is a graphical illustration of a person's preference between two or more goods. Figure 12 is an example of an indifference curve involving two goods. The subject concerned is as happy with point P1 (15 units of A and 4 units of B) as with point P2 (6 units of A and 10 units of B).

Information bias (*see under* Bias)

Informed choice (*see under* Subjective preference)

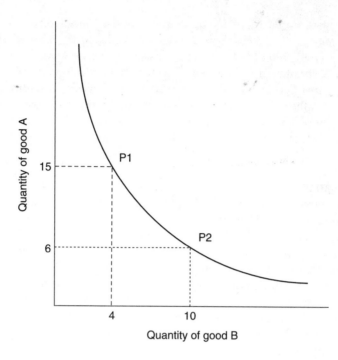

Figure 12 The concept of indifference

Intention to treat analysis

This is a method of analysis for randomized controlled trials whereby all patients randomly allocated to one of the treatments in a trial are analysed together irrespective of whether or not they completed or received that treatment. This is recommended to ensure that the benefits of randomization are not lost through introduction of biased selection at the analysis stage. Intention to treat analysis is also referred to as pragmatic trial or programme effectiveness analysis. This is to be contrasted with (i) **efficacy analysis** which compares outcomes only for subjects who have completed treatment with that intended at randomization (such an analysis is also referred to as an exploratory trial analysis or biological efficacy test analysis) and (ii) treatment received analysis which compares subjects according to which treatment they actually received irrespective of which treatment they were assigned to at randomization. This latter analysis is also termed 'as treated analysis' by some trialists and less kindly as 'garbage analysis' by other commentators (Newell DJ (1992) Intention to treat analysis: implications for quantitative and qualitative research. *International Journal of Epidemiology*. **21**: 837–41. Peduzzi P, Detre K, Wittes J, Holford T (1991) Intent to treat and the problem of cross-overs. An example from the Veterans Administration coronary bypass surgery study. *Journal of Thoracic and Cardiovascular Surgery*. **101**: 481–7). While intention to treat analysis is rather straightforward to apply when the outcome is discrete, with continuous outcomes the analysis requires imputation of data and how to deal with those who actually switched treatments is more problematic.

Interim analysis
When designing a clinical trial, there are often areas surrounded by much uncertainty. For example, in calculating the sample size of the trial, we require an estimate of the variance of the patients' responses and there may not be much prior knowledge about this and a rough estimate has to be made. In other situations, for ethical reasons, we may wish to terminate a trial early if a treatment appears to be obviously superior to another from the early data. To enable us to decide when to stop or whether recruitment has to be increased, we need to do an analysis which may not be the final planned analysis. This is termed an interim analysis. As such, it is a scientific inferential process which uses appropriate statistical methods and hence has to be planned for with decision rules defined prospectively at the trial design stage. Such interim analyses are usually conducted when there is clearly a lack of intended effect, emergence of serious unpredicted adverse effects or overwhelming efficacy results in life-threatening or severely debilitating illness. Unplanned interim analyses outside these situations should not be conducted as they interfere with the internal validity of the trial (Sankoh AJ (1995) Interim analyses: an FDA reviewer's experience and perspective. *Drug Information Journal*. **29**: 729–37).

Internal validity
Internal validity refers to whether conclusions drawn with respect to the specific population under study are valid. For example, in an observational study evaluating the significance of various potential risk factors for a particular disease, systematic differences in the characteristics of different groups pose a serious threat to its internal validity. In other words, an association which is identified between a risk factor and the disease may arise solely because the risk factor is associated with another, more significant one.

International Classification of Diseases

The *International Classification of Diseases* (ICD) is a system of disease classification which is regularly updated by the World Health Organization. The classification has its roots in the standard nomenclature for causes of death first proposed by W Farr (1807–83). The latest revision is the 10th (ICD-10), published by the WHO in 1992. The 21 disease categories are shown in Table 3 below.

Table 3 Disease categories in ICD-10

I	Certain infections and parasitic diseases
II	Neoplasms
III	Diseases of the blood and blood-forming organs and certain disorders involving the immune mechanism
IV	Endocrine, nutritional and metabolic diseases
V	Mental and behavioural diseases
VI	Diseases of the nervous system
VII	Diseases of the eye and adnexa
VIII	Diseases of the ear and mastoid process
IX	Diseases of the circulatory system
X	Diseases of the respiratory system
XI	Diseases of the digestive system
XII	Diseases of the skin and subcutaneous tissue
XIII	Diseases of the musculoskeletal system and connective tissue
XIV	Diseases of the genitourinary system
XV	Pregnancy, childbirth and the puerperium
XVI	Certain conditions originating in the perinatal period
XVII	Congenital malformations, deformations and chromosomal abnormalities
XVIII	Symptoms, signs and abnormal clinical and laboratory findings, not classified elsewhere
XIX	Injury, poisoning and certain consequences of external causes
XX	External causes of morbidity and mortality
XXI	Factors influencing health and contact with health services

(World Health Organization (1992) *ICD-10 – International statistical classification of diseases and related health problems*, 10th revision. WHO, Geneva.)

International Conference on Harmonization (see ICH)

J

Jarman index

The Jarman index or the Jarman underprivileged area score (UPA(8)) was developed to serve as a measure of UK general practitioners' workload. It has also been used as a proxy measure for deprivation in medical general practice research although such use has been criticized (Jarman B (1983) Identification of underprivileged areas. *BMJ.* **286**: 1705–9. Jarman B, Townsend P, Carstairs V (1991) Deprivation indices. *BMJ.* **303**: 523. Hippisley-Cox J *et al.* (1997) Effect of deprivation on general practitioners' referral rates. *BMJ.* **315**: 1465–7).

Judgement

A judgement is an explicit indication of a person's (judge's) critical appraisal of available evidence.

Judgement analysis

Judgement analysis refers to the methodologies associated with the modelling and statistical analysis of how human judgements are made. Multiple regression analysis forms the basis of much of the analysis (Cooksey RW (1996) *Judgment analysis: theory, methods and applications.* Academic Press, San Diego).

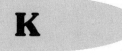

Keynes, John Maynard (1883–1946)

John Maynard Keynes was a British economist whose influential work led to the school of thought referred to as Keynesian economics. His book *The General Theory of Employment, Interest and Money* (1936) provided the framework for much of modern macroeconomic theory. His main thesis, unlike that of the **neoclassical economists**, was that self-correcting market forces were weak and that government intervention was necessary to control wide fluctuations and to ensure full employment.

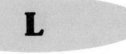

L

L'Abbé plot

This is a plot displaying individual trial results so that readers can rapidly identify which of the trials included in a systematic review show benefits in favour of the test treatment and which do not (Figure 13). The two axes of the plot represent the response of interest for the two treatment groups. Identical scales are chosen for each group's responses (y axis for test treatment and x axis for the control treatment) and the plane subdivided into two equal areas separated by a 45° diagonal line of equality. Therefore, trials which show results in favour of the test treatment fall in the region above the diagonal while those which favour the control treatment fall below the diagonal. The symbol (e.g. circles) chosen to represent the individual trial may be sized to reflect the sample size or inverse variance of the estimate and hence the weight which should be attached to each of the trials (L'Abbé KA, Detsky AS, O'Rourke K (1987) Meta-analysis in clinical research. *Annals of Internal Medicine.* **107**: 224–33).

Libertarianism (*see under* Utilitarianism)

Likelihood ratio

The likelihood of an outcome is the probability of its occurrence under a given probability model.

Likelihood = $p(y|\text{model})$

The likelihood ratio (LR) is simply the ratio of two likelihoods, i.e.

LR = $p(y|\text{model-1}) / p(y|\text{model-2})$

In Bayesian analysis, the likelihood ratio is used to transform the prior odds of one model compared to another, to the posterior odds as follows:

$p(\text{model-1}|y) / p(\text{model-2}) = \text{LR} \times [p(\text{model-1}) / p(\text{model-2})]$

Posterior odds = LR × prior odds

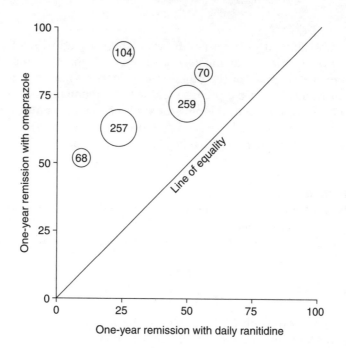

Figure 13 A L'Abbé plot

For a diagnostic test, the LR is the ratio of the probability of obtaining a result in subjects with the disease relative to the probability of obtaining the same result in subjects without the disease. Two likelihood ratios can be calculated in each clinical situation: (i) LR positive and (ii) LR negative, where LR positive is the ratio of the probability of obtaining a positive test result in diseased subjects relative to the probability of obtaining the same result in non-diseased subjects. The LR negative is the ratio of the probability of obtaining a negative test result in diseased subjects relative to the probability of obtaining the same result in non-diseased subjects.

Likert scale

The Likert scale, named after Rensis Likert, is also known as the summative scale. It is a rating scale based on the summative model, which assumes that individual items are monotonically related to the underlying attributes being measured and that the sum of the item scores is approximately linearly related to the attribute. The term is now used more loosely to describe any scale in which the items are scored on a categorical scale to show the degree of agreement, e.g. 1 = strongly approve; 2 = approve; 3 = neutral; 4 = disapprove; 5 = strongly disapprove.

Logic

Logic can be defined as the scientific evaluation of arguments where an argument is a group of statements, one or more of which are put forward to support one or more of the others. More succinctly, an argument is a statement which includes a premise and a consequential conclusion. The study of logic is aimed at developing the skills necessary for making sound arguments and for critically assessing those of others (Hurley PJ (1994) *A concise introduction to logic*. 5th edn. Wadsworth, Belmont, CA).

Logistic model

In many situations, we may wish to model the probability of a dichotomous outcome (e.g. dead or alive) as a function of several variables. The logistic model, defined by the equation below, is often useful.

$$\phi_i = \frac{1}{1 + e^{-\alpha_i'\beta}}$$

where ϕ is the probability of success for the ith group, α_i is a vector of known constants, α_i' is the corresponding transpose and β is a vector of unknown parameters which are to be estimated.

Logistic regression

A form of regression analysis used when the response (or dependent) variable is a dichotomous (binary, yes/no) variable. Suppose that the probability of an event which is dependent on a series of k variables (x or predictor variables) is given by p, then logistic regression takes the form:

$$\log_e \frac{p}{(1-p)} = \beta_0 + \beta_1 x_1 + \cdots + \beta_k x_k$$

where the β values are unknown coefficients to be estimated in the regression analysis.

Logistic transformation (see Logit)

Logit

Suppose that the probability of an event is p. The logit or **logistic transformation** is given by $\log_e \frac{p}{(1-p)}$. Such a transformation is useful, for example in expressing the logistic model in a linear form. Note that the logit model is a special case of the log linear model where the *y* variable is the odds and the link function is the log of an odds (*see under* **Odds ratio, Generalized linear model, Logistic regression**). (Bishop YM, Fienberg SE, Holland PW (1975) *Discrete multivariate analysis: theory and practice*. MIT Press, Cambridge, MA).

Log linear model
The log linear model is a special class of **generalized linear models** where the link function takes the form:

$$\log(y) = \alpha + \beta_1 x_1 + \cdots + \beta_k x_k$$

The α and β values are the coefficients to be estimated in such models. Note that *y* can take only positive values in such models (Agresti A (1996) *An introduction to categorical data analysis*. John Wiley, New York).

Longitudinal study (see *also under* Cohort study)
A study in which subjects are recruited and followed up forward in time, usually over many months or years. For example, in such a study, diabetic patients may be followed over a period of years to investigate how good blood glucose control affects the likelihood of complications, such as cataracts or peripheral neuropathy, developing.

Lorenz curve
The Lorenz curve is a useful graphical method, invented by a 19th century German statistician for depicting the distribution of income in a population. If one were to plot the cumulative proportion of total income versus the cumulative proportion of income recipients in a population, we would observe a straight line with unit slope, given perfect equality in income among individuals (Figure 14). The line will curve downwards if the income distribution is unequal and the more unequal the distribution, the further the curve will be from the diagonal (Brown WS (1995) *Principles of economics*. West Publishing Company, Minneapolis). The Lorenz curve can be used to calculate a coefficient of inequality, referred to as the **Gini coefficient**. This is the ratio of the area between the line of equality and the Lorenz curve (area A) and the area below the line of equality (areas A + B). The Gini coefficient has a useful quantitative economic interpretation. A value of 0.25 can be interpreted as meaning that if two incomes are drawn

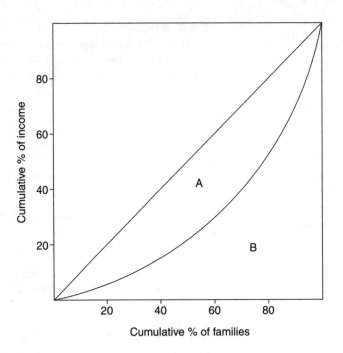

Figure 14 The Lorenz curve

at random from the population concerned, then the expectation is that on average the difference between them would be twice the value of the Gini coefficient multiplied by 100 (i.e. 50%) of mean income.

M

Macroeconomics

Macroeconomics is one of the two main branches (the other is microeconomics) of economic theory. It deals with the 'macro' or larger economic issues such as growth in **gross domestic product**, inflation and unemployment.

Main effect

In the analysis of the results of experiments, a main effect is a response caused by changing a single factor.

Malthus, Thomas Robert

Malthus was a British economist (1776–1834) who predicted poverty and starvation as inevitable consequences of the conflict between the laws of nature and human behaviour. He based his prediction on a model which assumed geometric growth in population and an arithmetic growth in food production. Fortunately, however, his prediction was wrong (Figure 15).

Managed care

In health services terminology, managed care refers to a variety of methods for managing the efficient delivery of comprehensive health care. Costs are contained through the control of the provision of services and the use of formularies while an attempt is made to maintain quality of care through careful clinical **audits**. The concept was developed in the United States in response to the escalating costs of health care and the perceived lack of accountability by the providers of health care. While there are many managed care structures, most fall into two categories: health maintenance organizations (HMOs) and preferred provider organizations (PPOs).

HMOs provide comprehensive managed health care in return for pre-payment. Such organizations may set up contracts with independent medical practices (independent practice association (IPA) model) to provide the services or hire their own salaried physicians (non-IPA or staff model).

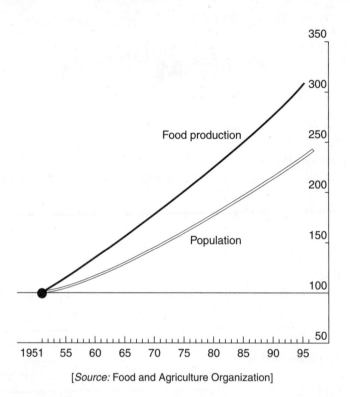

350

300

Food production 250

200

Population 150

100

50

1951 55 60 65 70 75 80 85 90 95

[*Source:* Food and Agriculture Organization]

Figure 15 Actual population growth and food production since 1951 (= 100%)

Independent doctors may organize themselves as independent groups to provide their services through the HMOs (group model). In return for guaranteed work, physicians agree to discounted payment and defined cost and quality controls.

The managed care system is still undergoing rapid evolution. The initial system consisting of little more than contracts with preferred providers is evolving into programmes keenly attuned to health outcomes, performance and league tables, and **medical informatics.** Patients within the managed care system are increasingly well informed and the delivery of care is being increasingly integrated across the primary–secondary care interface. Surprisingly, there has been little published on the systematic evaluation of the performance of the managed care organizations.

In Europe, the concept is applied to maximizing health gain of the community within limited resources. Close monitoring is undertaken to ensure that an appropriate range and level of services are provided within a framework of continuous improvement. National targets are set for both societal health and the meeting of individual health needs (Ingelhart JK

(1993) Managed care. *New England Journal of Medicine*. **327**: 742–7. Weiner J, de Lissovoy G (1993) Razing a tower of Babel: a taxonomy for managed care and health insurance plans. *Journal of Public Health Politics, Policy and Law*. **18**: 75–103).

Mann–Whitney statistic

In a comparison of two treatments, the Mann–Whitney statistic, denoted by $P(N>S)$, is an estimate of the probability that a randomly selected patient receiving a new treatment (N) would perform better than a randomly chosen patient receiving the standard treatment (S). For example, if 100 patients on treatment S were switched to the new treatment N and 80 got better and 20 got worse, then $P(N>S)$ is equal to 80/100 or 0.8. Ties are divided equally to contribute half a patient to each treatment. Calculation of $P(N>S)$ for results for a matched pair design is undertaken in a similar manner. Thus if 80 pairs show N to be better, $P(N>S)$ is again 0.8.

Estimates of $P(N>S)$ can be calculated directly from the raw data from two groups by calculating the proportion of all possible comparisons that favour N. For example, if n patients received N and s patients received S, then there are $n \times s$ or ns possible comparisons. The same calculation can be done using data from survival curves.

For continuous data, if we assume that the difference between the score of a randomly selected patient receiving treatment N and that of a randomly selected patient receiving treatment S is d, then $P(N>S)$ is an estimate of the probability that d is greater than zero. To calculate $P(N>S)$, the difference in the average scores for N and S is calculated and standardized by dividing by the standard deviation of this difference. The resulting standard normal score can then be converted to $P(N>S)$ from a standard normal table. For independent samples, the standard deviation is calculated as the square root of the sum of the variances of means of scores for N and S. Thus, if the standard normal score is 0 then $P(N>S) = 0.5$. If the standard score is 1.96 then $P(N>S) = 0.977$ (Colditz GA, Miller JN, Mosteller F (1989) How study design affects outcome in comparisons of therapy. I: Medical. *Statistics in Medicine*. **8**: 441–54).

Marginal cost (*see under* Incremental cost)

Marginal utility

Marginal utility refers to the change in utility resulting from the consumption of one additional unit of a good.

Market prices (*see under* **Gross national product**)

Markov chain (*see under* **Markov modelling**)

Markov chain Monte Carlo (MCMC) (*see under* **Markov modelling**)

Markov modelling

The Markov model, named after the 19th century Russian mathematician AA Markov, is often used in economic modelling, including pharmacoeconomic analyses. In Markov modelling, the Markov chain is used to represent recurrent events over time with the assumption that the probability of any future behaviour of the process, when its current state is known, is not altered by its more distant past behaviour. In health economics, Markov modelling is often used to simulate transitions to various health states.

To generate a Markov chain we sample from a conditional distribution:

$$x^{i+1} \sim p(x|x^i) \qquad \text{for } i = 1,2,\ldots$$

The literature now includes a very wide variety of applications of statistical modelling using numerical integration of the Markov chain (Markov modelling). The technique is often referred to as Markov chain Monte Carlo modelling (Metropolis N, Rosenbluth AW, Rosenbluth MN *et al.* (1953) Equations of state calculations by fast computing machine. *Journal of Physics and Chemistry*. **21**: 1087–91. Hastings WK (1970) Monte Carlo sampling methods using Markov chains and their applications. *Biometrika*. **57**: 97–109. Gilks WR, Richardson S, Spiegelhalter DJ (eds) (1996) *Markov chain Monte Carlo in practice*. Chapman and Hall, London).

Marshallian demand curve

The Marshallian demand curve is simply the curve showing the decrease in demand (x axis) with an increase in price (y axis). The area under the curve is often referred to as the ordinary or uncompensated or Marshallian consumer surplus (Marshall A (1920) *Principles of economics*. 8th edn. Macmillan, London).

Medicaid

A health care programme introduced in the USA in 1965 to reduce financial barriers to health care for certain low-income groups, with funding being provided jointly by the state and federal governments. The programme is administered independently by the individual states within broad federal guidelines (*see also* **Oregon plan**, an attempt by Oregon State to use cost benefit analysis to reform its programme).

Medical informatics

Medical informatics is the use and study of information science and technology in the delivery of health care. It calls upon other disciplines including mathematics, statistics, psychology, linguistics and philosophy. There is growing realization that to practise evidence-based medicine, practitioners need to acquire the ability to identify gaps in their knowledge and the means and skills to bridge those gaps. Given the explosion of medical information, the use of the best information science and technology to access the data efficiently is deemed to be essential by an increasing number of educationalists and policy makers.

Medical review criteria

Medical review criteria are systematically developed statements that can be used to assess the appropriateness of specific health care decisions, services and outcomes (Field MJ, Lohr KN (eds) (1990) *Clinical practice guidelines. Directions for a new program.* National Academy Press, Washington DC).

Medicare

A US federal government health insurance program introduced in 1965 to cater for individuals aged 65 and over and some groups of people with disabilities, notably patients requiring renal dialysis. As the US population ages, more resources are being consumed by this component of the health care system.

Medicinal product

A medicinal product is defined as (i) any substance or combination of substances presented for treating or preventing disease in human beings or animals or (ii) any substance or combination of substances which may be administered to human beings or animals with a view to making a diagnosis or to restoring, correcting or modifying physiological functions in human beings or animals (*see* Article 1 of Directive 65/65/EEC).

Medicines Commission

The Medicines Commission is an advisory body set up to advise the UK ministers of health on drug licensing issues. Applications for drug licences are evaluated by the Secretariat of the Medicines Control Agency with the advice of the Committee on Safety of Medicines (CSM). When a licence application is rejected, the drug manufacturer concerned can lodge an appeal to the Medicines Control Agency which is heard by the CSM with attendance by members of the Secretariat. If this appeal fails, the company concerned can further appeal to the Medicines Commission. If the advice of the MC is accepted by the UK ministers of health (the licensing authority) then the only other option open to the manufacturer is the court of law. In a recent case of licensing of a benzodiazepine, the CSM recommended recall of a licence, the MC reversed it and at the final stage, the licensing authority decided to adopt the CSM's advice. The case then went to the High Court.

Memphis indicators

A set of indicators used by health authorities in the UK for assessing the quality of prescribing by general practitioners. The indicators are: (i) the percentage of total costs accounted for by drugs of limited clinical value (e.g. cerebral vasodilators, antidiarrhoeals); (ii) the percentage of costs accounted for by selected modified-release preparations deemed to offer little advantage over conventional formulations (e.g. sustained-release non-steroidal anti-inflammatory agents and sustained-release salbutamol); (iii) the percentage of costs accounted for by selected combination products judged to be irrational or contributing little additional benefit relative to the single agents (e.g. diuretic-potassium combinations).

Merit good

A merit good is one whose consumption by others is regarded as useful and is encouraged by incentives, subsidy or coercion. An example is compulsory schooling or training.

MeSH thesaurus

MeSH is the abbreviation for Medical Subject Headings used in the thesaurus designed by the National Library of Medicine in Bethesda,

Maryland, USA. The thesaurus is used to create the *Index Medicus*, a directory of major scientific publications. The MeSH thesaurus has approximately 18 000 main subjects and is regularly updated. Table 4 gives the main subject classification.

Table 4 MeSH classification

A	Anatomy
B	Organism
C	Diseases
D	Drugs and chemical products
E	Analytical, diagnostic and therapeutic techniques and equipment
F	Psychiatry and psychology
G	Biological sciences
H	Physical sciences
I	Anthropology, education, sociology and social phenomena
J	Technology, industry, agriculture and food
K	Humanities
L	Information sciences and communication
M	Named groups
N	Health
Z	Geographical names

Meta-analysis

Meta-analysis refers to the systematic quantitative pooling of available evidence on a particular research question with the use of appropriate statistical methods. As such, it forms part of many systematic overviews. In the context of drug efficacy, clinical trial evidence is sought systematically and the relevant efficacy outcome data extracted. The data are then pooled using suitable weights such as sample variance or sample size. The pooled estimate of efficacy is then presented with the appropriate confidence bounds to define its precision. Although in medicine, meta-analysis is most widely used for pooling experimental data from randomized clinical trials (RCTs), observational data have also been meta-analysed. Methodology for incorporating observational data in meta-analyses of RCTs is also available but is not generally adopted.

Most meta-analyses are undertaken on the summary data reported in the individual trials being pooled and it is usually not possible to check on any inconsistencies. However, in certain circumstances, the records of the clinical trialists may be particularly good and the network exists for obtaining the individual patient data for revalidation (e.g. cancer clinical trial networks). A meta-analysis undertaken with revalidation and cross-checking of the individual patient data is called an individual patient meta-analysis.

Some authors use the term 'meta-analysis' synonymously with 'systematic overview' or 'systematic review' irrespective of whether statistical pooling is undertaken. Others, rather confusingly, use the term 'non-statistical meta-analysis' to refer to a systematic overview without statistical pooling.

Over recent years, clinical trialists proposing to undertake similar trials have started to design their studies to ensure that the results can be statistically pooled on completion. A meta-analysis of the resulting data is referred to as a prospective meta-analysis.

The results of a meta-analysis are usually presented graphically with confidence interval (typically 95%) estimates for the individual as well as the pooled estimates of effect (Figure 16).

In a meta-analysis, if the trials are arranged sequentially in order of publication date, it is possible to provide a pooled estimate for the first two trials and then to update this estimate with each subsequent trial. A meta-analysis undertaken with this approach is called a cumulative meta-analysis. The results of such a meta-analysis are shown in Figure 17 (Li Wan Po A (1996) Evidence-based pharmacotherapy. *Pharmaceutical Journal.* **256**: 308–12).

Meta-ethnography

Meta-ethnography is a method of analysis involving the comparative textual analysis of published qualitative field studies (ethnographies). In such an analysis, the approaches used are (i) combination of the individual ethnographies so that each can be presented in terms of the other; (ii) set against each other so that the basis of the refutation of one study by another can be made clear; (iii) linking of the individual studies to show how each informs or extends the others (Noblit GW, Hare RD (1988) *Meta-ethnography: synthesizing qualitative studies.* Sage Publications, Newbury Park).

Microeconomics

Microeconomics is one of the two main branches (the other being macro-economics) of economic theory. It deals with the 'micro' or small economic issues such as the behaviour of individual households, firms and industries.

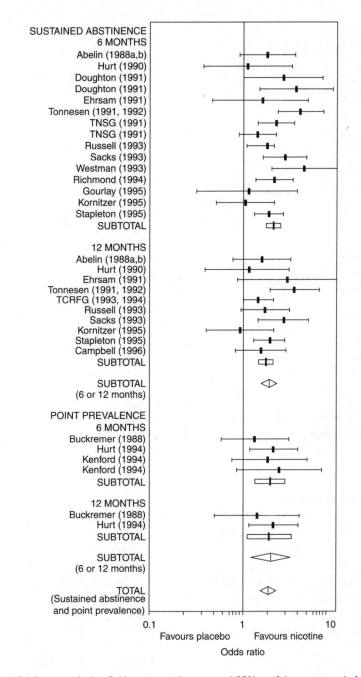

Figure 16 Meta-analysis: Odds ratios and associated 95% confidence intervals for effect of nicotine patch in smoking cessation

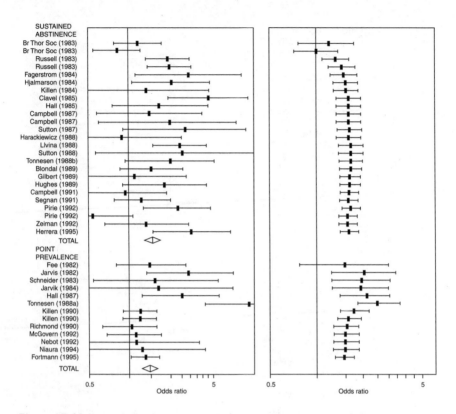

Figure 17 Meta-analysis: Comparison of conventional meta-analysis (left) and cumulative meta-analysis (right) of nicotine chewing gum in smoking cessation at 12 months. Odds ratios and associated 95% confidence intervals are shown

Model assessment

Model assessment refers to the validation of a mathematical model, in which the focus is on how well the model predicts the observations rather than how well it fits the data. In such an assessment, it is usual to replicate design points to estimate pure error and then estimate lack of fit by adding additional design points within the domain of the predictor (X) variables. Consider a simple straight line model of the form $Y = a X + b$ where Y is the response variable and a and b are the intercept and slope respectively. In estimating the coefficients of the model, Y values will be obtained for various X values. Replicates (repeat observations of Y at the same X value) are obtained to estimate the pure error. Y values corresponding to new X values, within the domain of the original X values, are obtained to test for lack of fit.

Monetary policy

The policy adopted by a government and/or a country's central bank (e.g. Federal Reserve in the USA and the Bank of England) with respect to money supply and interest rates in order to control inflation rate and employment.

Monopolistic competition

Monopolistic competition exists in a market when there are many sellers and yet because of customer loyalty, for example through brand loyalty, they have some influence over prices. They are therefore able to make some supernormal profits. This is in contrast to firms operating under pure competition when they are all price takers or to a firm operating as a monopoly or price setter.

Monopoly (see under Monopolistic competition)

Monopsony

A market situation where there is only one buyer. For example, in a country with a comprehensive national health service, the market for drugs is essentially monopsonistic. In contrast, a monopolistic market has a single supplier. With both monopolies and monopsonies, competition is imperfect and **allocative efficiency** is rare.

Monotonically related

Two variables are monotonically related if an increase in value in one variable leads to an increase or stabilization in the value of the other and vice versa. A monotonically increasing (decreasing) sequence is one in which the next value is always greater (smaller) than the previous value.

Monte Carlo simulation

A method for random sampling from defined probability distributions. Monte Carlo sampling is widely used for simulating physical systems such as queues, spatial distributions and drug responses. The method is also used for numerical integration, generally of complex functions which cannot be handled analytically.

Moral hazard

Moral hazard refers to the risk, faced by the insurer, of increased consumption of insured services by the insured because of the reduction in out-of-pocket price. More generally, a moral hazard exists whenever one party to a contract is able to use asymmetric information in a manner which adversely affects the other party. For example, a doctor may overtreat a patient to obtain a higher fee or a pharmacist may sell more drugs than a patient requires.

Morgenstern, Oskar (see von Neumann, John)

MOS 36-item short-form (see SF-36)

Multicolinearity

Multicolinearity is a problem which arises in the estimation of coefficients of a statistical model when the predictor variables are correlated. The regression coefficients are unstable in the presence of multicolinearity (i.e. small changes in the values of the predictor variables lead to large changes in the estimated coefficients) and are hence not reliable.

N

N of I trial

An N of 1 trial is a controlled trial in a single individual. Such a trial is usually randomized and double blind to minimize bias. It is usually used when the available evidence about a particular intervention is insufficient or cannot be applied to that individual. A standard design for an N of 1 trial is for the individual patient to take either the drug under study or a placebo in a randomized, double-blind manner for a pre-determined period of time. The effects are monitored and a second period of treatment undertaken in the same way. Periods of paired treatments can be repeated and conclusions drawn about the relative efficacy of the treatments (Guyatt GH, Keller JL, Jaeschke R *et al.* (1990) The n-of-1 randomised controlled trial: clinical usefulness. Our three year experience. *Annals of Internal Medicine.* **112**: 293–9).

National Co-ordinating Centre for Health Technology Assessment (NCCHTA)

The NCCHTA was established by the UK Department of Health in 1996 to manage, provide support to, develop and promulgate its health technology assessment programme. The Centre is a consortium which includes the Wessex Institute for Health Research and Development at the University of Southampton and the University of York's Centre for Health Economics and Department of Health Sciences and Clinical Evaluation (http://www.soton.ac.uk/~wi/hta/index.html).

National Institute of Clinical Excellence (NICE)

NICE is an institute being set up by the UK Department of Health to promote clinical cost-effectiveness and the production and dissemination of clinical guidelines (DoH (1997) *The new NHS.* Cmd 3807. HMSO, London).

National Schedule of Reference Costs

The National Schedule of Reference Costs are cost data which NHS trusts are required to publish in a consistent manner so that performance on efficiency can be bench-marked (DoH (1997) *The new NHS*. Cmd 3807. HMSO, London).

NCE

NCE is the abbreviation for new chemical entity in relation to drug licence applications to the US Food and Drug Administration.

NDA

NDA stands for new drug application in drug licensing terminology. In evidence-based medicine, NDA refers to number of deaths avoided. Let $F_1(t)$ and $F_2(t)$ be the risk of deaths observed in a trial with patients receiving treatments 1 and 2 respectively. The absolute risk reduction (ARR) is given by:

$$ARR = F_1(t) - F_2(t)$$

The number of deaths avoided is given by:

$$NDA = n \times ARR$$

where n is the number of patients receiving treatment 2. In some papers, the authors take n to mean the whole population to whom the results of the trial are being extrapolated.

Negative likelihood ratio

The negative likelihood ratio (NLR) is defined by the equation:

$$NLR = \frac{(1 - sensitivity)}{specificity}$$

The negative likelihood ratio indicates how much more (NLR > 1) or less (NLR < 1) likely a negative result is to be found in a person with the condition compared to one without (Correction (1998) *BMJ*. **316**: 225).

Neoclassical economics

Neoclassical economists built on the work of Adam Smith (classical school) and claimed that market forces were strong enough to overcome economic shocks and move back to equilibrium without government intervention. Society, they argued, has a natural social order. The neoclassical vision was much favoured until the great depression of the 1930s when the world economy plunged into deep depression and unemployment reached record levels. Despite this apparent failure of the neoclassical vision, many modern economists in fact call themselves neoclassicals.

Net national product (NNP) (see under Gross domestic product)

NHS (National Health Service)

The NHS is the organization which provides health care to the United Kingdom population. It was set up immediately after the Second World War to provide a comprehensive health service for all. 'Comprehensive' was defined as 'available to all people' and covering 'all necessary forms of care'. Despite a number of reforms, the system has operated successfully for over five decades (DoH (1946) *A national health service*. Cmd 6502. HMSO, London. DoH (1997) *The new NHS*. Cmd 3807. HMSO, London).

NHS Executive

The NHS Executive is part of the UK Department of Health, with a central office in London and in Leeds and eight regional offices spread across the country. The Executive provides managerial support to the NHS.

NHS trust

NHS trusts are public bodies within the UK National Health Service, responsible for providing hospital and community health care.

NNT

The NNT or number needed to treat is the term used to define the reciprocal of the risk or rate difference. In a comparative study of two treatments A and B, suppose that the number of patients cured after receiving treatments A and B are 80/100 and 60/100 respectively. Then the difference in rate of cure is equal to 20/100. The reciprocal of this value, 5, is the NNT. This is interpreted as 'on average 5 patients need to be treated with treatment A for one more patient to be cured than would be the case if they received treatment B'. The NNT applies to risk of harm too. Suppose that following treatment with A and B, the rates of headache in the two groups of 100 patients in the same trial were 20/100 and 15/100. The estimate difference in risk would be 5/100 to give a reciprocal or NNT of 20. In other words, treating patients with A instead of B would on average result in one more case of headache per 20 patients (*see under* **Risk reduction** and **Risk**).

Normal distribution

A random variable is one, say X, which follows the probability density distribution $f(x)$:

$$f(x) = \frac{1}{\sqrt{2\pi\sigma^2}} \exp(-\frac{1}{2}(\frac{x-\mu}{\sigma})^2), x \in \Re$$

where μ is the mean and σ^2 is the variance of the distribution.

The normal distribution is used to model many continuous variables such as weight, blood pressure and height.

If we have a normally distributed variable X with mean μ and variance σ^2 which can be written more simply as $N(\mu,\sigma^2)$ then any linear transformation of X such as $aX + b$ will also be normally distributed as follows $N(a\mu + b, a^2\sigma^2)$. A particularly useful transformation is to variable:

$$Z = \frac{X-\mu}{\sigma}$$

Z, which is called the **standard normal variate**, will be normally distributed with mean 0 and variance 1.

Normative economics (*see under* Positive economics)

Null hypothesis (*see* Hypothesis testing)

Number needed to treat (*see* NNT)

Number of deaths avoided (*see* NDA)

O

OBM (*see* **Opinion-based medicine**)

Odds ratio

The odds of an outcome (e.g. adverse reaction following exposure to a drug) is the ratio of the probability of the outcome occurring to the probability of it not occurring. If the odds (O) of an event occurring following exposure to drug A is (Oa) and the odds of the same event occurring following exposure to drug B is (Ob), the ratio of the two odds (Oa/Ob) is known as the odds ratio (OR).

In the above example, an odds ratio of, say, 5 means that the odds of having the event in question following exposure to drug A is five times that following exposure to drug B.

Table 5 Contingency table showing a hypothetical set of outcomes following treatment of two groups of 100 patients each with two treatments A and B

	Treatment A	Treatment B
Event present	15	5
Event absent	85	95
Total events	100	100

The odds of the event happening with treatment A = 15/85 and with treatment B = 5/95. The odds ratio of the event happening with treatment A relative to treatment B = (15/85 divided by 5/95) = 2.68. The **risk** of the event happening with treatment A = 15/100 and with treatment B = 5/100. The **risk ratio** of event occurring with treatment A relative to B = (15/100 divided by 5/100) = 3. The **risk difference** for the event happening with the two treatments being compared = (15/100 – 5/100) = 0.1. The **number needed to treat** = 1/risk difference = 10.

OECD

The Organization of Economic Co-operation and Development (OECD) is an organization of developed nations which produces a range of economic, including health care, statistics about member countries as part of its collaborative research and development programme.

Office of Health Economics

This is a pharmaceutical industry-funded organization based in London, UK. It produces a range of publications on health care economics and one of its most recent ventures is the publication of a health economics evaluation database (HEED). The database is updated monthly and is available on CD-ROM (http://www.abpi.org.uk/ohe/htm).

Office of National Statistics (ONS)

The Office of National Statistics (1 Drummond Gate, London SW1V 2QQ) was formed in 1996 from the merger of the Central Statistical Office (CSO) and the Office of Population Censuses and Surveys (OPCS), both of which were part of the UK Government Statistical Service. In addition to taking over all the functions of the CSO and OPCS, the ONS provides labour market statistics, a role previously undertaken by the Department of Employment. The ONS compiles data on the population's demographics, economic and health trends, financial statistics, industrial output and retail prices, among others. The ONS also undertakes an annual General Household Survey although this may well be discontinued following a current review.

Office of Population Censuses and Surveys

The Office of Population Censuses and Surveys (OPCS) was part of the Government Statistical Service and was responsible for conducting the national census. In 1996, the OPCS merged with the Central Statistical Office to form the Office of National Statistics.

Office of Technology Assessment (OTA)

The US OTA has as remit the evaluation of technology in its broadest sense, including health technology (http://www.wws.princeton.edu:80/~ota/).

Off-label use

Off-label use of medicines refers to their prescribing and use outside the licensed indications. This is a common practice in paediatrics and obstetrics since, for ethical reasons, trials are difficult to conduct in the subject groups concerned. Therefore, when the drug dossiers are submitted for licensing of the products concerned, manufacturers usually put in a disclaimer and in the absence of data, the licensing authorities are unable to make meaningful comments except those based on pre-clinical animal data.

Oligopoly (see under **Oligopsony**)

Oligopsony

An oligopsony is a market characterized by a few large buyers so that each needs to take careful account of the others' reactions when formulating their own purchasing strategies. In contrast, an oligopoly is a market characterized by a few large manufacturers or suppliers. Again, each needs to carefully consider the others' potential reactions when formulating their own pricing strategies. Just like monopolies, oligopolies exist only if there are sufficient barriers to prevent other firms from entering the market. Both technical and strategic barriers can exist (e.g. barriers to entry presented by branding or patents, both of which are important in the pharmaceuticals industry).

ONS (see **Office of National Statistics**)

OPCS (see **Office of Population Censuses and Surveys**)

Open-ended contingent valuation (see under **Contingent valuation**)

Operational research

Operational research is the use of qualitative methods for modelling complex systems in an environment of constraint, uncertainty and change so that a better understanding of those systems can be obtained and their solutions sought within the resultant structured framework. The aim of OR practitioners is to improve organizational performance through better decisions (*see also* **Decision analysis**).

Opinion-based medicine

Opinion-based medicine (OBM) is the use of expert or consensus opinion in the practice of medicine. This approach contrasts with **evidence-based medicine** which focuses on systematic evaluation of the available evidence. In practice, given that randomized controlled trials have answered only a few of the many clinically relevant questions, even the keenest EBM enthusiast will have to resort to OBM at least some of the time.

Opportunity cost

Opportunity cost refers to the value of goods and services foregone by not adopting the next best alternative. By adopting one alternative, one is foregoing the benefit to be derived from the next best alternative.

Oregon plan

This was an attempt by the US Oregon Health Services Commission to revise Oregon's Medicaid program through a cost benefit analysis of the various health services. The objective was to produce a priority list of services from which specific services could be chosen for coverage in order of their appearance in the list until the budget was exhausted. The initial rankings caused much controversy because many were clinically counter-intuitive. A notorious example of this was the higher priority assigned to dental caps for pulp exposure than to surgery for ectopic pregnancy. Revised rankings have since been produced (Eddy DM (1991) Oregon's methods. Did cost-effectiveness analysis fail? *Journal of the American Medical Association.* **266**: 2135–41).

Orthogonality

In statistical analysis, orthogonality is said to exist when there is no correlation between the experimental levels of the predictor variables and the effects of the various variables can be estimated independently.

Outcome measure (see Outcomes)

Outcomes

Any measure of health status used in monitoring patients in observation or intervention trials. The narrower term 'endpoints' refers to health events that lead to completion or termination of follow-up of a subject in a health study (e.g. death or a myocardial infarction).

Overhead cost

The cost assigned to resources which are used in the production of goods or services but which cannot readily be attributed to the production of one particular good or service (e.g. heating and lighting, and administrative support).

P

PACT data

PACT or Prescription Analysis and Cost data is an approach introduced in 1988 by the UK Department of Health to disseminate information to individual general practitioners about their own prescribing patterns in relation to that of others. The data can be used by doctors to audit their own prescribing. By doing so, the Department hoped that general practitioners would be made aware of the costs of drugs and thereby be encouraged to prescribe more thoughtfully (DoH (1987) *Promoting better health*. HMSO, London).

Quarterly feedback is provided to general practitioners by the national Prescription Pricing Authority (PPA) which collates all the data. Several levels of detail can be provided ranging from top-line information to detailed brand-specific analyses. Unfortunately, because diagnoses are not attached to prescriptions, the PPA data cannot in general be used to audit appropriateness of prescribing. Inferences can only be drawn about issues such as proportion of generic to branded products prescribed and ratios of corticosteroids to beta-agonists prescribed in asthma (*see under* **ASTRO-PU** and **STAR-PU**).

PACTLINE

PACTLINE is an electronic link between health authorities in Great Britain and the Prescription Pricing Authority which allows the former to download computerized data about general practice prescribing in their areas (Majeed A, Evans N, Head P (1997) What can PACT tell us about prescribing in general practice? *BMJ*. **315**: 1515–19).

Palliative care

Palliative care is defined by the World Health Organization (WHO) as the active total care of patients whose disease is not responsive to curative treatment. Palliative care aims to provide the best possible quality of life for patients and their families through management of their psychological, social and spiritual well-being. According to the WHO, palliative care, which has its roots in the hospice movement, (i) affirms life and regards dying as a normal process; (ii) neither hastens nor postpones death; (iii) provides relief from pain and other distressing symptoms; (iv) integrates the psychological and spiritual aspects of patient care; (v) offers a support system to help patients live as actively as possible until death; (vi) offers a support system to help the family cope during the patient's illness and in their own bereavement (WHO (1990) *Cancer pain relief and palliative care.* WHO Technical Report Series 804. World Health Organization, Geneva).

Paradigm

A paradigm is made up of the general assumptions, laws and techniques used by members of a particular scientific community. The paradigm defines what is acceptable within the science which it governs. Kuhn popularized this concept (Kuhn T (1970) *The structure of scientific revolutions.* Chicago University Press, Chicago) in his explanation of the way science develops. He defines a pre-science phase when research activity within a given field is disorganized and diverse. This then becomes more directed and structured (the normal science phase). During this phase, scientists develop further explanations but come across difficulties and falsifications of laws and assumptions underlying the existing paradigm. A crisis develops when controversy gets out of hand. With new theories to resolve the crisis, a new normal science phase is re-established before the next crisis is encountered. The work of Copernicus, for example, led to a paradigmatic change. Commentators are suggesting that the wide acceptance of evidence-based medicine is leading to a paradigm change in clinical practice.

Paradox of thrift (*see under* Fallacy of composition)

Pareto criterion

The Pareto criterion, based on a suggestion made by Vilfredo Pareto, states that a change can be said to be an improvement only if it makes at least one person better off without making another worse off (Pareto V (1906) *Manual of political economy.* (Schwier AS, Page AN (eds)) Macmillan, London).

Pareto efficiency (*see under* Efficiency)

Pareto improvement

A Pareto improvement is one by which at least one person is made better off while no one is made worse off.

Pareto optimality

A situation is said to be Pareto optimal if no one can be made better off without making another person worse off. Pareto optimality is often used as a reason for maintaining the status quo and is criticized for this.

Patient outcomes research team (PORT)

The patient outcomes research team programme was established in 1989 by the Agency for Health Care Policy and Research of the US Department of Health and Human Services to organize and fund researchers to resolve the diagnosis and treatment of common conditions such as angina, cataracts and prostate disease. PORT teams are usually made up of clinicians, assisted by scientists such as biostatisticians.

Patient's expected event rate

The patient's expected event rate (PEER) is the probability that the patient will experience the event concerned (e.g. myocardial infarction) over the time frame considered. Estimates of PEER are ideally obtained from robust prognosis papers. However, in practice it may be necessary to obtain PEER from historical controls. PEER is used for calculating number needed to treat (**NNT**) from reported **odds ratios** as follows:

$$NNT = \frac{1 - (PEER) \times (1 - OR)}{(1 - PEER) \times (PEER) \times (1 - OR)}$$

Patients' preferences (see Utility)

PEER (see Patient's expected event rate)

Perceived substitute effect

This is used to describe the effect which the perception that a product can be satisfactorily substituted by another has on price sensitivity (Nagle TT,

Holden RK (1994) *The strategy and tactics of pricing: a guide to profitable decision making*. 2nd edn. Prentice-Hall Inc, Englewood Cliffs).

Performance measures

Performance measures are methods or instruments used to estimate or monitor the extent to which actions of a health care practitioner or provider conform to practice guidelines, medical review criteria or standards of quality (Field MJ, Lohr KN (eds) (1990) *Clinical practice guidelines: directions for a new program*. National Academy Press, Washington DC).

Period prevalence (*see under* Incidence)

Personal Social Services

Personal Social Services are services in the United Kingdom for vulnerable people, including those with special needs because of old age or physical or mental disability, and children in need of care and protection. Examples are the services provided by social workers, residential care homes for the elderly, meals on wheels and homes for the mentally handicapped.

Perspective

In economic analyses, perspective refers to the viewpoint adopted in the analysis. Ideally, in an economic analysis, a societal perspective should be adopted but more commonly the perspective of a specific funding agency (e.g. the National Health Service or a hospital trust) is used.

Perverse taste paradox (*see* Utilitarianism)

Pharmaceutical alternatives

The US Food and Drug Administration defines pharmaceutical alternatives as drug products which contain the same therapeutic moiety but are different salts, esters or complexes of that moiety or are different strengths or dosage forms for which there are no data available to make assessments of **bioequivalence**.

Pharmaceutical care

Pharmaceutical care is a term used to define patient-centred, outcomes-oriented pharmacy practice. The objective is to optimize the patient's health-related quality of life. Close professional interaction with the patient and other health care workers is necessary so that health may be promoted, disease prevented and therapy monitored effectively (APA (1995) *Principles of pharmaceutical care.* American Pharmaceutical Association, Washington).

Pharmaceutical equivalents

The US Food and Drug Administration defines pharmaceutical equivalents as drug products which contain the same active ingredient(s), are of the same dosage form and route of administration and are identical in strength or concentration. They are formulated to meet compendial or other applicable standards but may differ in shape, appearance, excipient composition, expiration time and labelling.

Pharmaceutical Price Regulation Scheme (see PPRS)

Pharmacokinetic-pharmacodynamic modelling

For many drugs, the blood level is linearly related to the intensity of its pharmacological and/or clinical effects, which can be both beneficial and toxic. For other drugs this cannot be applied so readily. For example, the liver toxicity of paracetamol is non-linear with respect to blood level in that the drug is not toxic to the liver below a threshold level but toxicity is severe above it. Pharmacokinetic-pharmacodynamic modelling (PK-PD modelling) attempts to define the precise relationship between the kinetics of a drug's distribution and the kinetics of its pharmacological effects (Smith RB, Kroboth PD, Juhl RP (eds) (1986) *Pharmacokinetics and pharmacodynamics.* Harvey Whitney Books, Cincinnati. Cutler NR, Sramek JJ, Narang PK (1994) *Pharmacodynamics and drug development.* John Wiley, Chichester).

Pharmacokinetics

Pharmacokinetics is the study of the distribution of drugs in the body as a function of time. Such studies are important for working out appropriate dosage regimens for individual drugs so that efficacy can be optimized and toxicity minimized.

Pharmacotherapy

Pharmacotherapy is the term used to describe treatment undertaken with drugs (pharmacological agents).

Phase I studies (see Drug development)

Phase II studies (see Drug development)

Phase III studies (see Drug development)

Phase IV studies (see Drug development)

PK-PD modelling (see Pharmacokinetic-pharmacodynamic modelling)

Point prevalence (see under Incidence)

Poisson distribution

The random variable X representing the number of events $(x = 0, 1,..)$ occurring by time t in a **Poisson process** with mean rate λ has a Poisson distribution with parameter λt as described in the following equation:

$$P(X = x) = \frac{e^{-\lambda t} (\lambda t)^x}{x!}$$

The Poisson distribution can be used to model distribution of events not only in time but also in space. It has been used to model the occurrence of adverse drug reactions. The mean and variance of a Poisson distribution are both given by $\mu = \lambda t$.

The Poisson distribution is an approximation to the **binomial distribution** $B(n, \frac{\mu}{n})$ where n is the number of trials and $\frac{\mu}{n}$ is the probability of success in each trial.

Poisson process

A Poisson process is one in which events occur spontaneously, at random, in time. Many phenomena of biological or medical interest can be modelled using the Poisson process (e.g. number of accidents per day). A Poisson process is specified by three postulates: (i) the probability of an event occurring during any small interval $(t, t + \delta t)$ is equal to $(\delta t) \lambda \delta t + o(\delta t)$

where λ is the mean rate, t is the time and $o(\delta t)$ is a value which tends to zero as the small time interval tends to zero; (ii) the probability of more than one event occurring during a small interval is equal to $o(\delta t)$; (iii) the occurrence of events after any time t is independent of the occurrence of events before time t. The Poisson process described above is referred to as being stationary because of the assumed constant mean rate. The process can be extended to model more complicated processes such as by using mean rates which vary with time (non-homogeneous Poisson process).

Population at risk

The population at risk denotes the denominator in the calculation of event (e.g. death, disease or adverse reaction) rates in epidemiological studies. For example, when calculating the death rate for a particular community, the population at risk is usually taken as the estimate of the population of that community thought to be alive on July 1 of the calendar year concerned. In estimating the incidence rate of an adverse drug reaction, the population at risk is the number of patients exposed to the drug and observed for the adverse reaction.

PORT (see Patient outcomes research team)

Positive economics

Positive economics is an approach to economic analysis which is only concerned with the consequences of different changes or policies and does not make judgements about the desirability of alternative allocation of resources. This is in contrast to normative economics which is concerned with analysing the desirability of different changes and policies. Normative economics is also referred to as 'welfare economics'. The normative approach is used when criteria are required to rank different options (Johansson PO (1991) *An introduction to modern welfare economics*. Cambridge University Press, Cambridge).

Positive rate of time preference (see under Discounting)

Post-randomization consent design

In a conventional randomized controlled trial (RCT), informed consent is sought from patients to participate in the trial. Those who agree to

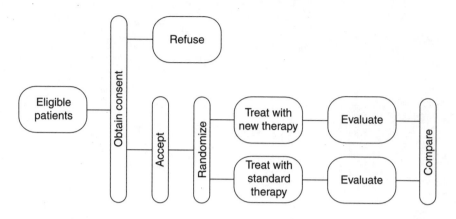

Figure 18 Pre-randomization consent design

participate are then randomized to receive, in a two-armed trial, the test treatment or the control, which is chosen to be the best standard therapy (Figure 18). In the conventional RCT, recruitment of patients is often difficult as the need to obtain prior consent before randomization often deters patients and doctors. Zelen suggested randomizing patients to the different treatment groups prior to seeking consent. Such a design is referred to as a post-randomization consent design or alternatively a pre-consent randomization or randomized consent design. In such a trial the group randomized to receive the best standard therapy is not bothered further except that it is evaluated and its outcomes compared to those of the other treatment groups. Those randomized to the treatment group are then asked for consent to participate in the trial and be given the test treatment. Those who agree receive it and those who refuse obtain the best standard therapy. The outcome of the three groups can then be compared (Figure 19). An extension of this design is the double randomized consent design in which consent is sought from both groups after randomization (Figure 20).

The use of these randomized consent designs has caused much controversy among ethicists, statisticians and clinical trialists. The main concern is that proper informed consent is not obtained from at least some of the patients although the double randomized consent design overcomes some of this problem. Note, however, that in such trials double blinding is not possible and introduction of substantial bias is possible (Altman DG, Whitehead J, Parmar MKB *et al.* (1994) Randomized consent designs in cancer trials. *European Journal of Cancer.* **31**: 1934–44).

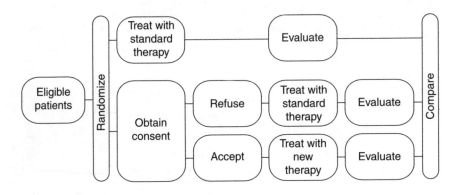

Figure 19 Post-randomization consent design I

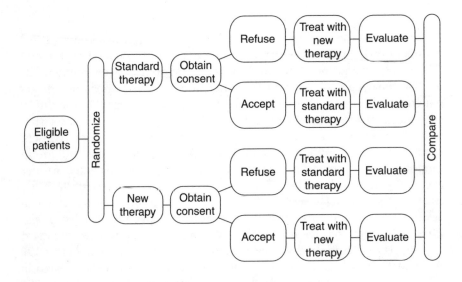

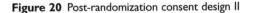

Figure 20 Post-randomization consent design II

PPRS

The Pharmaceutical Price Regulation Scheme (PPRS) is a system introduced in 1957 by the UK Department of Health (DoH) to regulate drug prices and the profits of the pharmaceutical industry. Each year, pharmaceutical companies supplying drugs to the NHS are required to make financial returns to the DoH, which assesses the information to ensure that prices, profits and costs are within acceptable limits. Historically, profits of about 20% are deemed reasonable and aggregate expenditure on sales promotion is limited to 9% of total sales. For comparison most large established pharmaceutical companies spend about 10% of total sales on research and development. The PPRS system is meant to be voluntary but clearly the perceived penalty attached to non-acquiescence ensures that most companies adhere to the scheme. The complexity of transfer pricing by multinationals makes this system difficult to police. The Public Accounts Committee reviews the agreement at regular intervals. There is much controversy about the value of PPRS. The UK government would point out that its application has led to a thriving pharmaceutical industry but others have argued that it is a disincentive to investment in research and development (Green DG, Brown P, Burstall ML *et al.* (1997) *Should pharmaceutical prices be regulated?* Institute of Economic Affairs, Health and Welfare Unit, London).

Practice guidelines
Practice guidelines are systematically developed statements to assist practitioner and patient decisions about appropriate health care for specific clinical circumstances (Field MJ, Lohr KN (eds) (1990) *Clinical practice guidelines: directions for a new program.* National Academy Press, Washington DC).

Pragmatic trial (see under Intention to treat analysis)

Pre-certification
Pre-certification refers to the system whereby clinicians, usually within a **managed care** system, must seek permission to provide specific services to patients before initiating such treatment.

Pre-consent randomization design (see under Post-randomization consent design)

Prescribing analysis and cost data (see PACT data)

Prescription Drug User Fee Act 1992
The Prescription Drug User Fee Act 1992 (PDUFA) is a US law which authorizes the US Food and Drug Administration to levy user fees on

manufacturers who submit licence applications to the agency. The objective was to generate additional funding to eliminate the backlog of applications and speed up approval time for new drug and biological applications. The aim was to complete the review of 90% of priority applications within six months and standard applications within 12 months. A recent review indicates that the approval time for user fee drugs was considerably shorter than for non-user fee drugs – 14.5 versus 31 months (Prescription Drug User Fee Act 1992. Public law 102–571 (October 29, 1992); 21 USC 379; 106 Stat 4491. Kaitin KI (1997) The prescription user fee act of 1992 and the new drug development process. *American Journal of Therapeutics*. **4**: 167–72).

Price sensitivity
Price sensitivity refers to how sensitive sales of a product are to changes in price. Unlike **price elasticity**, price sensitivity is a qualitative concept (Nagle TT, Holden RK (1994) *The strategy and tactics of pricing: a guide to profitable decision making*. 2nd edn. Prentice-Hall Inc, Englewood Cliffs).

Primary care
Primary care has recently been defined as the function of providing 'integrated, accessible health care services by clinicians who are accountable for addressing a large majority of health needs, developing a sustained partnership with patients, and practising in the context of family and the community' (Donaldson MS, Yordy KD, Lohr KN, Vaselow NA (eds) (1996) *Primary care: America's health in a new era*. National Academy Press, Washington).

Primary care groups
Primary care groups (PCGs) are a new organizational entity announced by the UK government in its 1997 White Paper on proposed reforms of the National Health Service (DoH (1997) *The new NHS*. Cmd 3807. HMSO, London). The PCGs will unify the budgets and management of teams of general practitioner (GP) practices and are intended to replace health authorities and individual GP fundholders. The PCGs will have the opportunity to become freestanding **primary care trusts**. The government's intention is for each PCG to contain up to 50 GPs from as many as ten practices and typically cover populations of 100 000.

Primary care trusts (see under Primary care groups)

Primary outcome measure

In a clinical trial, a primary outcome measure is a prospectively defined outcome which the investigators consider to be of primary importance. Such an outcome can then be used to define the sample size of the trial and to define clinically meaningful changes on which to base judgements as to whether a treatment is effective or not. Such outcome measures can be supplemented with secondary outcome measures. The latter can be used to support the conclusions to be drawn from the primary outcomes or to generate new hypotheses. 'Primary and secondary outcome measures' are also used in meta-analyses.

Primary–secondary care interface

The interface between health care workers employed in hospitals on the one hand and general practice on the other.

Prisoners' dilemma

The prisoners' dilemma is a classic scenario in game theory used to illustrate how independent decision making can lead to inferior results for the parties involved. Similar scenarios are widely used to illustrate decision making by players in an oligopoly (a market dominated by a few firms which have to consider each other's possible retaliatory actions) (Gibbons R (1992) *A primer in game theory*. Harvester Wheatsheaf, Hertfordshire).

Private goods (see under Public goods)

Probabilistic functionalism

Probabilistic functionalism is an approach suggested by Egon Brunswik for studying and modelling human judgement (Brunswik E (1955) Representative design and probabilistic theory in a functional psychology. *Psychological Review*. **62**: 193–217). The approach is based on two propositions: (i) that the chief task of psychology is to understand how an individual functionally relates to his or her environment; (ii) that the relationships are stochastic or based on probabilistic relationships.

Probability of superiority estimate

In a comparative study, the probability of superiority estimate (PS) is the probability that a randomly sampled patient from a population given a test treatment will have a superior outcome to that of a randomly sampled patient from a population given the control treatment.

$$PS = p(y_1 > y_2)$$

An unbiased estimate of PS is given by U/n_1n_2 where U is the Mann–Whitney statistic and n_1 and n_2 are the sample sizes for the two groups. The PS is an attractive method for expressing comparative efficacy of two interventions. Note, however, that it requires dichotomizing continuous response data and defining when a treatment is superior to another, which may not always be easy (Grissom RJ (1994) The probability of superiority of one treatment over another. *Journal of Applied Psychology.* **79**: 314–16. Colditz GA, Miller JN, Mosteller F (1988) The effect of study design on gain in the evaluation of new treatments in medicine and surgery. *Drug Information Journal.* **22**: 343–52).

Standardizing the continuous data to the standard normal deviate Z has been proposed (*see* Effect size and Appendix in Colditz *et al.* referred to above). PS has also been called the **common language effect size** in this context (McGraw KO, Wong SP (1992) A common language effect size statistic. *Psychological Bulletin.* **111**: 361–5).

$$Z = \frac{(\bar{y}_1 - \bar{y}_2)}{\sqrt{(s_1^2 + s_2^2)}}$$

The PS is then the area to the left of the Z value under the standard normal curve. Thus, if the Z value is 1.645, the PS = 0.95. If Z = –1.645 then the PS = 0.05.

If a series of PS values are available from k trials then a pooled PS can be obtained by first obtaining a pooled Z value:

$$Z_p = \frac{\sum z}{\sqrt{k}}$$

A sample weighted pooled Z score ($Z_{ps} = \dfrac{\sum n_i z_i}{\sqrt{n_i^2}}$) can be obtained and the corresponding PS read from the appropriate standard normal table.

PS scores can be derived from a range of other statistics. If the *t* values and sample sizes are given in a two-treatment comparison then:

$$Z_p = -\frac{t}{\sqrt{n}}$$

If the sample sizes are not equal then:

$$Z_p = -t\frac{\sqrt{(\frac{s_1^2}{n_1} + \frac{s_2^2}{n_2})}}{\sqrt{(s_1^2 + s_2^2)}}$$

If Glass's or Hedges' effect size is used, PS is estimated using the following conversion:

$$PS = 0.7071ES$$

Production possibility frontier

A production possibility frontier is a boundary which defines what can be produced given factor of production constraints (financial budget or labour units) and prior choice of what to produce. Figure 21 illustrates the

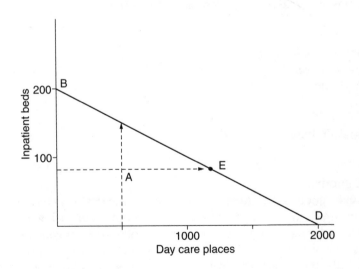

Figure 21 Production possibility frontier

concept using as an example the allocation, by a health authority, of a $1m budget to two competing claims: provision of day care places or hospital beds for mentally ill patients. Each day care place costs $500 while a hospital bed costs $5000. With the allocated budget, the health authority can provide 2000 day care places or 200 beds. Line BD, the production possibility frontier, shows the alternative, allocatively efficient combinations, such as point E, of day care and hospital beds which can be provided. Point A, on the other hand, is not efficient since day care places can be increased without decreasing hospital beds and vice versa.

Production possibility frontiers or curves need not be linear and can be generalized to deal with more than two choices (Phelps CE (1997) *Health economics*. 2nd edition. Addison Wesley, Reading, USA).

Prognosis
The likely clinical progress of a patient or disease over time.

Programme effectiveness analysis (see Intention to treat analysis)

Prospective case-control study (see under Case-control study)

Prospective meta-analysis (see under Meta-analysis)

Prospective study (see also under Cohort study)
A prospective study is one in which subjects are recruited and followed forward in time.

Protopathic bias (see under Bias)

Public goods
Pure public goods are those which are characterized by collective property rights from which no one can be excluded. Examples of such goods are air quality and sunlight. Those goods are not traded in any organized market. These goods can be separated from quasi-private goods and pure **private goods**. With the latter, individual property rights are assigned, potential customers can be excluded and the goods are traded competitively and

freely. Examples of such goods are houses and cars. **Quasi-private goods** are similar to private goods except that they are not freely traded in competitive markets. Examples are public libraries and park amenities (Mitchell RC, Carson RT (1989) *Using surveys to value public goods: the contingent valuation method.* Resources for the Future, Washington DC).

Public interest detailing (see **Academic detailing**)

Publication bias
The bias which arises when positive results are published while negative or null results are not (*see* **File drawer problem** and **Funnel plot**).

Purchasing power
The purchasing power of a currency (PPC) is the amount of goods that it will purchase in its home economy. A conversion rate between currencies can therefore be based on what one currency unit (e.g. US$) will buy in its home economy (the USA) and working out how many currency units (e.g. Yen) would be required in another country (Japan) to buy the same amount of goods. The US$ is often used as the reference currency unit for such comparisons. A PPC-based conversion rate is therefore not the same as the market rate as the former takes account of cost of living in the different countries. However, a key component of international economic analysis is the theory of purchasing power parity which says that in the long run, a US$ should purchase as much in the USA as anywhere else in the world after adjustment for transportation costs and therefore, in the long run, changes in exchange rates reflect relative inflation rates. Economic statistics such as the **gross domestic product** (GDP) are often reported in terms of both market rates and PPC.

Use of PPC produces some surprising rankings. For example, in the World Bank report for 1995, while the USA has the highest world GDP at both PPC and market exchange rates, China moves from seventh position based on market exchange rates to second position using PPC. India similarly moves from 15th position to fifth position. The PPC is often referred to as the purchasing power parity in the popular literature.

Q

QALY

Few treatments are free from side-effects. Indeed, in some areas of therapy (e.g. cancer chemotherapy), the side-effects (e.g. nausea and alopecia) may be so distressing that patients may refuse therapy. When assessing the effectiveness of such treatments it is therefore important to take account of both the positive and the adverse effects. In other words, the outcome (e.g. survival time or life-years gained) is quality adjusted to take account of the overall impact of treatment on the patient. Such quality-adjusted or utility-adjusted gains in life-years are called QALYs (Figure 22). The gain in quality-adjusted life-years following effective treatment is as shown. The weighting to be used for quality adjustments is controversial. A commonly cited weight matrix is that developed by Rosner and Watts (*see* **Rosner and**

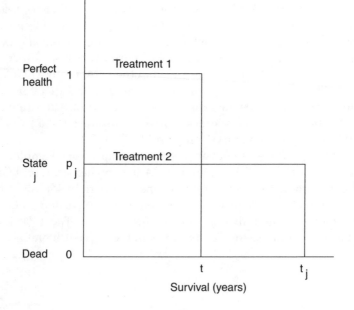

Figure 22 QALY

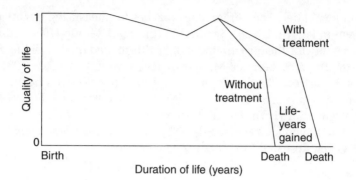

Figure 23 QALY gained

Watts matrix). This was developed on a small sample of some 70 subjects (doctors, nurses, patients and healthy volunteers) and there is therefore concern about the generalizability of the results. Other concerns with QALYs are that (i) as commonly used, they relate to point estimates whereas marginal cost curves tend to turn upwards and marginal benefit curves tend to turn downwards as the programme size increases; (ii) the weights used depend on specific social preferences and the common assumption of cross-cultural generalizability is unlikely to be valid. Figure 23 illustrates the concept of life-year gained. (McDowell I, Newell C (1966) *Measuring health: a guide to rating scales and questionnaires.* 2nd edn. Oxford University Press, Oxford).

Q-TWiST analysis

In Q-TWiST analysis, prolongation of life brought about by treatment is quality adjusted to take account of the time spent without symptoms or toxicity (*see under* **QALY**).

Quality of Life (QoL)

Quality of life refers to the broad construct which reflects both subjective and objective judgements about issues which impinge on the total well-being of individuals including health, social, environmental and spiritual aspects. In health care, we are usually interested only in the health-related issues. Various instruments are available for measuring health-related quality of life (HRQoL) to yield values which can then be used to adjust length of life in order to account for the negative impact which ill health can have on such things as physical and mental function, perception and social opportunities. The different approaches for measuring quality of life are shown in Figures 24–26. (*See* **QALY**) (EuroQoL Group (1990) EuroQoL – a new facility for the measurement of health-related quality of life. *Health Policy.* **16**: 199–208. Bergner M, Bobbit RA, Carter WB *et al.* (1981) The sickness impact profile: development and final revision of a health status measure. *Medical Care.* **19**: 787–805. Ware JE, Sherbourne CD (1992) The MOS 36-item Short-Form Health Survey (SF-36). *Medical Care.* **30**: 473–83. Hunt SM, McEwen J, McKenna SP (1981) *The Nottingham health profile user's manual.* Galen Research Consultancy, Manchester).

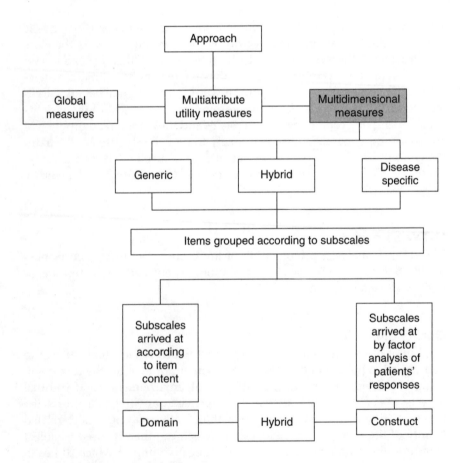

Figure 24 Measuring quality of life I

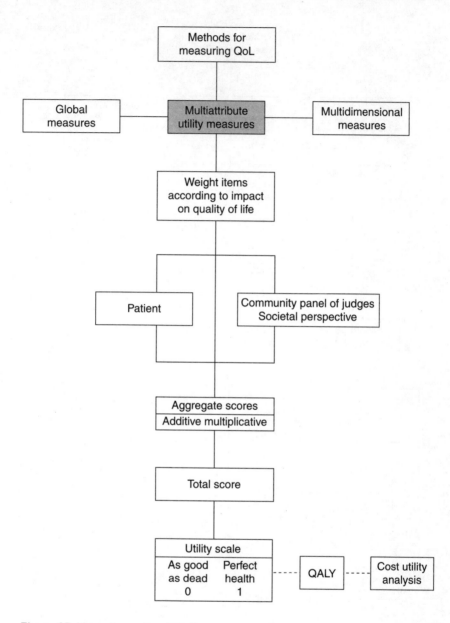

Figure 25 Measuring quality of life II

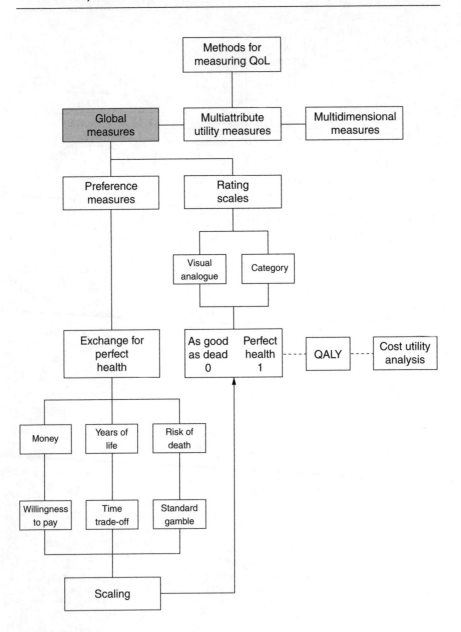

Figure 26 Measuring quality of life III

Quality standards (see Standards of quality)

Quantal response data

Quantal response data are dose-response data for which the response is an all-or-nothing phenomenon (e.g. dead or not, cured or not, impaired or not, etc.). An alternative term is quantal assay data. For example, in the testing of an antibiotic, we may administer different doses to several groups of people and observe how many people develop diarrhoea in each group, thus providing us with quantal data (Morgan BJ (1992) *Analysis of quantal response data.* Chapman and Hall, London).

Quasi-private goods (see under Public goods)

R

Randomized clinical trial (*see under* **Clinical trial**)

Randomized consent design (*see under* **Post-randomization consent design**)

RCT (*see under* **Clinical trial**)

Reactance theory
Reactance theory was put forward to explain why people often do the opposite to what they have been asked to do. The theory suggests that people believe they have a set of free behaviours in which they can engage. Any threat to these generates a reaction aimed at preserving the threatened free behaviours. The individual demonstrates an intensity of reactance, which is in proportion to the magnitude of the perceived threat, the number of free behaviours being threatened and the value placed on the intensity of the reactance on them. Reactance theory has been used to explain non-compliance to prescribed treatment regimens (Fogarty JS (1997) Reactance theory and patient noncompliance. *Social Science and Medicine.* **45**: 1277–88. Brehm JW (1966) *A theory of psychological reactance.* Academic Press, New York).

Read codes
The Read codes are a clinical classification system being developed by the UK Department of Health for computerizing medical records and, in particular, general practice data. The intention is to produce comprehensive information about individual patients so that clinical decisions can be better informed. The data should also allow better audit of health needs and hence better targeting of health care resources (DoH (1990) *New classification will streamline computerized medical records.* DoH, London. Smith N, Wilson A, Weekes T (1995) Use of Read codes in development of a standard

data set. *BMJ.* **311**: 313 –15. Information Management Group (1993) *A national thesaurus of clinical terms in Read codes.* HMSO, London. Information Management Group (1993) *What are Read codes?* HMSO, London. Information Management Group (1993) *Read codes and the terms project: a brief guide.* NHS Management Executive, London). The future of the Read codes has recently been called into question as a result of a critical report (February 1998) by the UK National Audit Office. The report has called for an urgent independent evaluation into whether further investment would be justified and whether the codes were usable in a clinical environment.

Table 6 Structure of the Read codes

Preferred term: diabetes mellitus
Synonym: sugar diabetes
Abbreviation: DM
Cross-referencing

Read	Clinical term (30 and 60 character term shown)	ICD-9	ICD-10
B200	Diabetes mellitus	250	E10-E14
B2001	Diabetes mellitus with no complications	250-0	E13
B2003	Diabetes mellitus with neuropathy	250-3	E13
B2003	Diabetes mellitus with nephropathy	250-5	E13
B2004	Insulin-dependent diabetes mellitus	250	E10
B2005	Non-insulin dependent diabetes	250	E11
B2006	Malnutrition-related diabetes mellitus	250	E12

Recall bias (*see under* Bias)

Receiver operating characteristic (ROC) curve
The ROC curve is a plot of the values for the sensitivity of a diagnostic test against the corresponding (1-specificity) values. Such curves are useful for examining the discriminatory ability of markers of disease or of diagnostic tests. A major problem with ROC curves is that they lead investigators to choose cut-offs which arbitrarily classify patients as diseased or not and hence do not allow subsequent workers to choose alternative cut-offs under different circumstances, such as greater limitation of resources (Swets JA, Pickett RM (1992) *Evaluation of diagnostic systems: methods from signal detection theory.* Academic Press, New York).

Recognition lag

The recognition lag is the time it takes for policy and decision makers to recognize that a policy change is necessary (*see* **Impact lag** and **Implementation lag**).

Reference pricing

Reference pricing refers to the use of a reference drug from a particular therapeutic class to calculate the reimbursement to be made for any drug belonging to that category dispensed by third parties. Such schemes are usually adopted by prescription pricing agencies to control drug costs. Therefore the reference drug is usually the cheapest in the category concerned unless a case can be made for the use of a more expensive alternative based on **cost-effectiveness analysis**.

Relative income hypothesis

The relative income hypothesis (*see also* **Absolute income hypothesis**) postulates that the distribution of income in a society affects the individual's risk of mortality (Gravelle H (1998) How much of the relation between population mortality and unequal distribution of income is a statistical artifact? *BMJ.* **316**: 382–5).

Relative price effect

The relative price effect is the change in the unit cost of a government-provided good or service relative to the general price level.

Relative risk (*see under* Risk)

Relative risk reduction (*see under* Risk reduction and Risk)

Residual error

The residual error is the difference between an observed value and the value predicted by a statistical model. For example, consider a linear regression model of the form $y = ax + b$, where x is the predictor variable, y is the response variable and a and b are constants. If a set of y values are observed at different x values, the coefficients a and b can be estimated from the paired x and y values. For any new x value, we can obtain a predicted y value from the straight line equation. The difference between that value and the observed value is the residual error.

Resource intensity weights

Resource intensity weights are weights developed to capture the intensity of resource utilization by individual **case mix groups** (Baladi JF (1996) *A guidance document for the costing process*. Canadian Coordinating Office for Health Technology Assessment, Ottawa. http://www.ccohta.ca).

Response expectancy

The effect of patients' prior expectation of the efficacy of treatments being evaluated on their observed responses to those treatments. For example, it has been observed that when patients are administered a placebo, if they are told to expect an active treatment, then their response is different to that seen when they are told that they will receive either an active treatment or a placebo. Similarly, the design of a study may affect response rate, a phenomenon probably partially attributable to response expectancy (Kirsch I, Weixel LJ (1992) Double-blind versus deceptive administration of a placebo. *Behavioural Neuroscience*. **102**: 319–23. Colditz GA, Miller JN, Mosteller F (1988) The effect of study design on gain in the evaluation of new treatments in medicine and surgery. *Drug Information Journal*. **22**: 343–52).

Retrospective study

A study which is undertaken after the patients have been enrolled and using data on events of interest which have already occurred. Epidemiological studies are generally of this type (*see* **Case-control study**).

Risk

Risk may be defined as the probability of an adverse event multiplied by the severity of the loss which experiencing that event would entail. More generally, the risk of an event is simply defined as the probability of that event occurring following exposure to the risk factor. The absolute risk is given by the incidence of the event. Therefore it requires both a numerator and denominator to calculate and is quantified on a probability scale (0 to 1). If we administer a particular antidiabetic agent to, say, 100 patients and observe that five develop diarrhoea, then an estimate of the risk of diarrhoea developing is given by 5/100 or 0.05.

Risk can also be expressed as a conditional probability. For example, the risk of cervical cancer (CC) in women receiving unopposed hormonal replacement therapy (HRT) can be written as $P(CC|HRT) = p$ where p is the incidence of CC in this group of patients.

Risk can be expressed in relative terms, for example risk of developing a particular adverse event among individuals exposed to a drug compared to those not exposed. If the risk (or incidence) of the event in those exposed is Re and that in the non-exposed group is Ro, the ratio (Re:Ro) is known as the risk ratio or relative risk (RR).

Suppose that there are n individuals in a comparative trial of two treatments A and B and that the outcomes with respect to an adverse event are as shown in Table 7 with all the tabular entries as integers.

Table 7 Calculation of relative risk from data in a contingency table

	Treatment A	Treatment B	Total
Adverse event present	a	c	a+c
Adverse event absent	b	d	b+d
Total	a+b	c+d	a+b+c+d = n

The relative risk (RR) or risk ratio of the event occurring with treatment A relative to B is given by:

$$RR = \frac{a/(a+b)}{b/(c+d)}$$

An RR value of 5 means that the event is five times more likely to occur in the exposed group than in the non-exposed group. In pharmacoepidemiological studies investigating association between an adverse reaction and a drug, for example, the larger the RR value, the stronger the association. Values close to unity suggest no relationship and negative values suggest a negative or protective effect (e.g. intake of foods high in antioxidant compounds and cardiovascular disease). RR can only be calculated in a cohort or experimental study.

The risk difference (RD) or **risk reduction** is given by:

$$RD = \frac{a}{a+b} - \frac{c}{c+d}$$

(*see under* **Risk reduction**).

Risk difference (see under Risk)

Risk ratio (see under Risk)

Risk reduction

In assessing and attributing risk, it is best to express the risk relative to a control (see under **Risk**). For example, in estimating by how much an antibiotic reduces the risk of traveller's diarrhoea, we could observe 100 patients receiving it and report how many (say five) develop diarrhoea. The estimate of absolute risk of diarrhoea would be 5/100 or 0.05. This figure, however, does not tell us by how much the antibiotic has reduced the incidence of diarrhoea. To do this, we may study a control group of patients given a placebo to obtain another estimate of risk of diarrhoea for this group of patients (say 10/100 or 0.1). The difference in the two rates (0.05) gives us an estimate of the risk reduction in absolute terms. For this reason this value is called the absolute risk reduction (ARR). On average, five fewer patients out of 100 treated would develop diarrhoea than if they received a placebo.

The reciprocal of the risk reduction gives us the number needed to treat (see **NNT**), 20 in this instance. The NNT tells us that on average 20 patients need to be given antibiotics for one more patient to be protected from diarrhoea when compared to placebo.

The risk reduction may also be expressed as a proportion or percentage of the risk in the control group to produce a relative risk reduction (RRR), expressed as a proportion or percentage. In the above example, the relative risk reduction is given by (0.1 – 0.05)/0.10 or 0.5. Expressed as a percentage the RRR is 50%. This appears more impressive than the ARR of 0.05 or 5%.

It is worth noting that, perhaps confusingly, both the absolute and the relative risk reduction terms are relative to a control group. The terms used refer to how the values are expressed. The RRR is as a proportion or percentage of the control rate or risk while the ARR is on its own.

Root mean square error

The root mean square error (RMSE) is an estimate of the standard deviation associated with experimental error. For a sample of n observations $x_1, x_2,...,x_n$, the root mean square error or standard deviation is defined as:

$$RMSE = \sqrt{\frac{1}{n-1}(x_i - \bar{x})^2}$$

Rosner and Watts matrix

This is a disability-distress matrix (see below) developed by Rosner and Watts giving weights or utilities for quality-adjusted life-years gained as a result of a particular intervention (Rosner).

Table 8 The Rosner and Watts disability-distress matrix

Disability	None	Mild	Moderate	Severe
			Distress	
None	1.000	0.995	0.990	0.967
Slight	0.990	0.986	0.973	0.932
Severe	0.980	0.972	0.956	0.912
Severely limited performance	0.964	0.956	0.942	0.870
No paid employment or education	0.946	0.935	0.900	0.700
Chair-bound	0.875	0.845	0.680	0.000
Bedridden	0.677	0.564	–	–1.486
Unconscious	–1.028	–	–	–

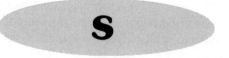

S

Scarcity

Scarcity is often referred to as the fundamental economic problem because human wants are unlimited. It can be argued that without scarcity there is no need to trade off alternatives and hence no need for economics as a discipline.

Secondary care

Secondary (health) care refers to specialist care, typically provided in a hospital setting or following referral from a primary or community health professional.

Secondary outcome measures (see under Primary outcome measures)

Selection bias (see under Bias)

Sensitivity

The sensitivity of a diagnostic test is the true positive ratio, that is, the proportion of patients with disease (D) who return a positive test ($+T$).

Sensitivity = true positive = $P(+T|D)$

Sensitivity analysis

Sensitivity analysis is the term used for describing recomputation of results using different parameter values or perspectives to investigate whether any conclusions drawn are altered as a result. Such analysis is particularly popular in the economic assessments of medical interventions, including pharmacotherapy. For example, in a cost-effectiveness analysis, the investigator may vary the estimates or probability of treatment failure to check whether cost-effectiveness rankings are sensitive to such changes. A sensitivity analysis undertaken to define the boundaries where the conclusions drawn change qualitatively is called a *threshold analysis*. For example, a treatment may be more cost-effective than another provided the relapse rate remains below 10% but the ranking is changed at higher relapse rates.

SF-36 form

The SF-36 form is an instrument developed to measure health status and is for use in clinical practice and research, health policy evaluations and general population health surveys. Also referred to as the Medical Outcomes Study (MOS) 36-item short-form, it assesses, through multi-items subscales, eight health concepts: (i) limitation in physical activity through ill-health; (ii) limitations in social activities because of emotional problems; (iii) limitations in usual role activities through physical health problems; (iv) bodily pains; (v) general mental health, including psychological stress and well-being; (vi) limitations in usual role activities resulting from emotional problems; (vii) vitality (energy and fatigue); and (viii) general health perceptions (Ware JE Jr, Sherbourne CD (1992) The MOS 36-item Short-form Health Survey (SF-36) I. Conceptual framework and item selection. *Medical Care*. **30**: 473–83).

Shared care

The co-ordinated care of patients across the primary (community or general practice) and secondary (hospitals) health care interface.

Shared care protocol

Consensus protocols for the clinical management of patients across the primary (community or general practice) and secondary health care interface. These generally deal with issues such as the prescribing of expensive or problematic drugs (e.g. use of cytotoxics and luteinizing hormone-releasing hormone analogues).

Short-form 36 (see **SF-36 form**)

Side-effect

A side-effect of a drug is any positive or negative effect which is not the intended therapeutic effect. Pharmacovigilance experts recommend abandoning this term but given its wide acceptance, this is unlikely to happen.

Significance level

When setting up a hypothesis test, we start off by formulating a **null hypothesis** (H_0). In frequentist or classic statistics, we postulate a probability model such that the difference in effect between two treatments would be normally distributed with mean zero and a variance which we would estimate from the sample drawn. We also postulate an alternative hypothesis (H_1), such that the difference in mean is not zero. This alternative hypothesis will be accepted if the null hypothesis is rejected based on a previously set level of error which we would be prepared to accept. This error level (**Type 1 error**), relating to rejecting the null hypothesis when it is in fact true, is the significance level of the test. Sometimes the probability of a particular observation under the probability model postulated under H_0 is also referred to as the significance level.

Smith, Adam (1723–90)

Adam Smith, a Scot, is widely regarded as the father of modern economics. His book, *An Enquiry into the Nature and Causes of the Wealth of Nations*, published in 1776, is looked upon by many economists as the most influential book on economics ever written. His main thesis was that if each person were free to pursue his or her own interests, then nature would guide the economy as if it was an 'invisible hand' and there was no need for government intervention. Progress, he argued, would result from new technology and the specialization of labour. His ideas were further developed by others to lead to the school of thought now popularly referred to as the classical school.

Societal perspective

In analysing the impact of a health care intervention, the perspective adopted will affect the outcome and it is generally accepted that a societal perspective, which takes account of the effect on the social welfare of everyone, is preferable. In such an analysis, all medical and non-medical costs and all personal indirect costs, irrespective of who pays, are included. Health prevention strategies which show up poorly when more restricted perspectives are used, often show up quite well when this societal perspective is adopted.

Specificity

In diagnostic testing, the specificity is the proportion of subjects without disease who test negative.

Specific rate

Specific rate is the frequency of a particular event (death, adverse reaction, disease, etc.) in a particular subset of the population. Examples of commonly used specific rates are age-specific rates and cause-specific rates. For example, infant mortality which is expressed as an age-specific rate (e.g. 10 per 1000 population) is often used as an index of quality of health care in comparative studies. Matrices are often used to simultaneously represent age-and disease-specific death rates.

Staging bias (see under Bias)

Standard deviation

The standard deviation is a measure of the spread of a distribution and is equal to the square root of the **variance**. If the distribution is Gaussian (or normal) then the mean ± 1.96 standard deviation is expected to cover 95% of the measurements. The standard deviation of a population is normally referred to by the letter sigma (σ) and that of a sample by the letter (s).

Standard error

The standard error (SE) is the standard deviation of a statistical *estimator* such as the mean or a regression coefficient. The standard error of the mean (SEM) is, for example, a widely used statistic as it describes the precision associated with the estimate of the mean. The standard error is equal to the standard deviation of the individual measurements divided by the square root of the sample size.

Standard gamble

The standard gamble is a method for estimating the utility of a particular outcome from a particular perspective. Judges are asked to choose between life in a particular known health state and a gamble with a probability p of obtaining complete cure and a probability $(1-p)$ of death. The probability p is altered until the judges have no preference for either state. The probability p is then a measure of the preference or utility for the health state.

Standard normal variate

The standard normal variate, commonly referred to as Z, is a normally distributed variable with mean zero and variance 1 (*see under* **Normal distribution**).

Standardized mortality rate

The standardized mortality rate is a mortality rate adjusted to take account of the composition of the population to which it refers.

Standards of quality

Standards of quality are authoritative statements of (i) minimum levels of acceptable performance or results; (ii) excellent levels of performance or results; (iii) the range of acceptable performance or results (Field MJ, Lohr KN (eds) (1990) *Clinical practice guidelines: directions for a new program.* National Academy Press, Washington DC).

STAR-PUs

When undertaking comparisons of prescribing trends across different regions of a country, simple averages and proportions can be highly misleading because it is well known that the elderly, for example, require medication more frequently than the young. Therefore, doctors serving areas with a higher proportion of elderly patients would be expected to prescribe more. The STAR-PU (or specific therapeutic group age-sex related prescribing unit) is a weighting scheme developed to make some of the necessary adjustments before cost comparisons are made at the therapeutic group level (*see* **ASTRO-PUs.** Lloyd DCEF, Harris CM, Roberts DJ (1995) Specific therapeutic age-sex related prescribing units (STAR-PUs): weightings for analysing general practices' prescribing in England. *BMJ.* **311**: 991–4).

State-transition model

The state-transition model is a dynamic mathematical model which assigns individuals from a population to different categories or health states at recurring time intervals with defined transition probabilities. The model is often used to obtain estimates of life expectancy or quality-adjusted life expectancy. A state-transition model which assumes that the transition probabilities are dependent only on the current state is called a **Markov model** (Krahn MD, Mahoney MH, Eckman J *et al.* (1994) Screening for prostate cancer. A decision-analytic view. *Journal of the American Medical Association.* **272**: 273–80).

Stochastic model

A stochastic model is one which uses randomly generated data or parameters from particular probability distributions to describe a system, usually for predictive purposes. For example, in modelling patient through-put at a hospital pharmacy or clinic, the build-up of queues may be stochastically modelled by a computer simulating the arrival of patients by sampling from a **Poisson distribution** and the service time by sampling from an *exponential distribution*. Such a model can be used, for example, to predict the number of servers which would be required based on what would be judged to be acceptable waiting times. With computers, it is relatively easy to simulate even highly complex events such as the time spent by a **cohort** of patients in different health states (*see* **State-transition model**). In contrast, models which do not take account of the randomness of data and/or parameters by simulation are called deterministic models. These may be based on simple algebraic formulae such as number of servers required equals average number of patients arriving during the day divided by average number of patients which one pharmacist or doctor can attend to. Alternatively, differential equations may be used to describe the system being modelled. Such deterministic models are often used in pharmacokinetic studies although stochastic modelling is being increasingly used too, particularly when making predictions about individuals from population data. Note that precision estimates can still be made for predictions based on deterministic models provided we are willing to make assumptions about the precision or probability distribution of the input data.

Studentized value
A value which has been standardized by dividing it with its associated error to yield a dimensionless score. Thus the standardized residual is the residual divided by the estimated **standard deviation** of that residual.

Subjective preference
In the context of clinical trials or choice of treatment, subjective preference describes the choice of a particular treatment based on hunch, advice from friends or relatives or similar types of information. This is to be contrasted with informed choice when patients base their preferences on reliable estimates of risks and benefits from reliable data such as those derived from robust clinical trials or systematic overviews. However, irrespective of which approach is used, patients' preferences are often highly variable particularly when there are (i) major differences in possible outcomes; (ii) major differences between treatments in the range, likelihood and severity of outcomes; (iii) choices involving trade-offs between short- and long-term outcomes; (iv) choices involving a small probability of a major

adverse outcome; (v) only small apparent differences between the different options (Kassirer JP (1994) Incorporating patients' preferences into medical decisions. *New England Journal of Medicine.* **330**: 1895–6).

Surrogate outcome measure

A surrogate outcome measure is an end point used in lieu of another which is usually clinically more meaningful, but practically more difficult, to measure. For example, bone mineral density is often used as a surrogate outcome measure for bone fracture in clinical trials of prophylatic treatments, such as of hormone replacement therapy.

Survival analysis

Survival analysis refers to the study of time to events (e.g. time to death or recovery, time to failure of light bulbs, time to breakdown of a machinery component, etc.). The methodology overcomes problems associated with single time point estimations of failure (e.g. deaths, breakdowns and disease relapse) because the complete survival or failure curve is considered including **censoring** or loss to follow-up and end of study before 100% failure (*see* **Cox model, Censoring**). (Parmar MKB, Machin D (1995) *Survival analysis.* John Wiley, Chichester. Kalbfleisch JD, Prentice DL (1980) *The statistical analysis of failure time data.* John Wiley, New York).

Survival function

The survival function, usually written as $S(t)$, is the probability that the individual concerned survives longer than time t and hence is alive (or free from event) at time t. This can be calculated as follows:

$$S(t) = 1 - \int_0^t \phi(u)du$$

where $\phi(t) = \underset{\Delta t \to 0}{Limit} \{ \frac{P(death, \tau \to \tau + \Delta t)}{\Delta t} \}$

Symmetric distribution

A symmetric distribution is one in which values are symmetrically distributed around the mean. The population mean and median are then the same and the interval between the 25th percentile and the mean is equal to the interval between the mean and the 75th percentile. The Gaussian or **normal distribution** is an example of a symmetric distribution.

Systematic overview (*see under* **Systematic review**)

Systematic review

A systematic review or overview is a review of a particular subject undertaken in such a systematic way that the risk of bias is reduced. The review objectives are defined precisely and formal and explicit methods are used to retrieve the available evidence as comprehensively as possible. Inclusion and exclusion criteria for studies are defined. In the evaluation of medical interventions, outcomes to be used for efficacy or safety are identified and the relevant data extracted using explicit methods. Appropriate statistical methods are used for pooling any suitable quantitative data (meta-analysis) to provide an estimate of efficacy or safety and the clinical significance of the results discussed (Li Wan Po A (1997) A practical guide to undertaking a systematic review. *Pharmaceutical Journal*. **258**: 518–20).

T

TDM (see Therapeutic drug monitoring)

Technical efficiency (see under Efficiency)

Therapeutic drug monitoring (TDM)

For certain drugs such as gentamicin, blood levels need to be maintained within a certain range (often called a therapeutic window) to avoid inefficacy (associated with inappropriately low levels) and side-effects (associated with blood levels which are too high). To do this, blood levels of the drugs concerned are measured at intervals (i.e. subjected to therapeutic drug monitoring) and dosing regimens are altered if necessary.

Therapeutic equivalents

The US Food and Drug Administration (FDA) defines therapeutic equivalents as drug products which are pharmaceutical equivalents which can also be expected to have the same clinical effect and safety profile when administered to patients under the conditions specified in the labelling. The FDA classifies products as therapeutic equivalents if they meet the following criteria:

- they are approved as safe and effective
- they are pharmaceutical equivalents in that they

    (a) contain identical amounts of the same active drug ingredient in the same dosage form and route of administration, and

    (b) meet compendial or other applicable standards of strength, quality, purity and identity

- they are bioequivalent in that

    (a) they do not present a known or potential bioequivalence problem and they meet an acceptable *in vitro* standard, or

(b) they do present such a known or potential problem but have been shown to meet an appropriate bioequivalence standard

- they are adequately labelled

- they are manufactured in compliance with current good manufacturing practice regulations.

Therapeutic substitution

Therapeutic substitution, also referred to as therapeutic exchange or therapeutic interchange, refers to the dispensing of a drug of different chemical structure to that ordered by the prescriber because it is deemed to be therapeutically equivalent and/or more cost-effective. Therapeutic interchange has been used for H_2 antihistamines, quinolone antibiotics and tetracyclines. Just like generic substitution, it is a method for controlling drug costs (Rich DS (1989) Experience with a two-tiered therapeutic interchange policy. *American Journal of Hospital Pharmacy.* **46**: 1792–8).

Threshold analysis (*see under* Sensitivity analysis)

Time preference

Time preference refers to people's preference to consume now rather than in the future, everything else remaining constant. This provides the rationale for **discounting** future benefits.

Total phase

In the terminology of procedures associated with the marketing approval of therapeutic drugs by licensing authorities, the total phase refers to the interval between submission of an investigational new drug application (IND) and its marketing authorization by the appropriate regulatory agency (Food and Drug Administration in the USA, European Medicines Evaluation Agency in the European Community).

Total purchasing

In the context of UK health care, total purchasing refers to the purchase of hospital and community care services not covered by the **fundholding** scheme, by groups of general practitioners (GPs). The purchasing is done on behalf of patients by the GPs but the responsibility remains with the relevant health authority. This activity is being transferred to **primary care groups** (DoH (1997) *The new NHS*. Cmd 3807. HMSO, London).

Treatment guidelines (see under **Practice guidelines**)

Treatment received analysis (see **Intention to treat analysis**)

True negative ratio (see **Specificity**)

True positive ratio (see **Sensitivity**)

Type A adverse reaction

A type A (augmented effect) adverse drug reaction is one which is predictable from the pharmacology of the drug (e.g. hypotension caused by antihypertensive drugs and anticholinergic adverse effects of H_1 antihistamines). Such adverse reactions can usually be managed through appropriate dose titration. In theory, everyone is susceptible to type A reactions if the offending drug dose is increased sufficiently (Park K, Pirmohamed M, Kitteringham NR (1992) Idiosyncratic drug reactions: a mechanistic evaluation of risk factors. *British Journal of Clinical Pharmacology and Therapeutics*. **34**: 377–95).

Type B adverse reaction

A type B (bizarre) reaction is one which is idiosyncratic and usually appears to be independent of both dose and pharmacology of the drug. It is difficult to predict and is often serious. Examples are penicillin allergy and blood dyscrasias associated with some drugs (Park K, Pirmohamed M, Kitteringham NR (1992) Idiosyncratic drug reactions: a mechanistic evaluation of risk factors. *British Journal of Clinical Pharmacology and Therapeutics*. **34**: 377–95).

Type C adverse reaction

A type C adverse reaction is one associated with long-term therapy. Although the mechanism may be unclear, because such reactions (e.g. benzodiazepine dependence) are well described and are characteristic of drug classes, they can be predicted with reasonable degrees of certainty (Park K, Pirmohamed M, Kitteringham NR (1992) Idiosyncratic drug reactions: a mechanistic evaluation of risk factors. *British Journal of Clinical Pharmacology and Therapeutics*. **34**: 377–95).

Type D adverse reaction

This term is sometimes used to describe carcinogenicity and teratogenicity. There is usually a long delay between drug exposure and appearance of the adverse effect (Park K, Pirmohamed M, Kitteringham NR (1992) Idiosyncratic drug reactions: a mechanistic evaluation of risk factors. *British Journal of Clinical Pharmacology and Therapeutics*. **34**: 377–95).

Type I error

In hypothesis testing this is the probability of rejecting the null hypothesis when it is in fact true. This is a false-positive rate since it gives the probability of erroneously pronouncing a test significant. This error rate is often called the α error rate. Conventionally, the α rate in hypothesis testing is often set at 0.05 (Li Wan Po A (1998) *Statistics for pharmacists*. Blackwell Science, Oxford).

Type II error

In hypothesis testing the type II error is the probability of failing to detect an effect when it is in fact present. This error rate is often referred to as the β error. The complement of type II error (1-β) is called the power of the test. Conventionally, the β error is often set at 0.8.

U

Unique value effect

This term is used to describe the effect of unique attributes of a product on the price which purchasers are willing to pay. This is taken into account when pricing the product (Nagle TT, Holden RK (1994) *The strategy and tactics of pricing: a guide to profitable decision making*. 2nd edn. Prentice-Hall Inc, Englewood Cliffs).

Utilitarianism

Utilitarianism in the context of resource allocation is the philosophical approach which postulates that the greater benefit to society must be at the centre of all welfare states. This is in contrast to **libertarianism** which promotes the greatest good for the individual. To illustrate, consider the scenario shown in Table 9 which gives the success rates and costs of two different interventions for the same condition. For simplicity assume that failure will leave the patient in the same state.

Table 9 Utilitarianism versus libertarianism

	Cost per treatment	Number of patients	Total cost of treatment	Number of successes	Probability of success
Treatment A	£ 500	120	£60 000	30	0.25
Treatment B	£1500	40	£60 000	20	0.50

The utilitarians will adopt treatment A (overall more successes) while the libertarians will adopt treatment B (probability of success for the individual higher with treatment B). Most health authorities adopt a utilitarian approach in health care resource allocation. However, this approach is open to legal challenge. For example, in the UK in a recent case of the management of multiple sclerosis with interferon, the courts found that it was unlawful for a health authority to withhold giving the drug to a patient on the basis that the resources were needed elsewhere to treat more patients. The utilitarian approach may also lead to the treatment of what many regard as self-inflicted conditions (e.g. sexually transmitted diseases) in preference to, say, the rarer genetic diseases, a result referred to as the perverse taste paradox. Cases of doctors withholding heart surgery for smokers, on the basis that the resources would be better spent elsewhere, have also attracted much controversy (Mills JS (1962) *Utilitarianism*. Fontana, London. Entwistle V, Bradbury R, Pehl L *et al.* (1996) Media coverage of child B case. *BMJ*. **312**: 1587–90).

Utility

The concept of utility has its roots in the philosophy of **utilitarianism**, closely associated with the work of the 18th century philosopher Jeremy Bentham. He described utility thus: 'By utility is meant that property in any object whereby it tends to produce benefit, advantage, pleasure, good or happiness or to prevent the happening of mischief, pain, evil or unhappiness to the party whose interest is considered' (Bentham J (1990) *Introduction to the principles of morals and legislation*. Athlone Press, London, first published 1789).

Generally, utility can be defined as the benefits derived from consumption. Utility as proposed by Pareto, for example, is considered to be something personal and therefore non-comparable between persons (*see under* **Efficiency**). However, over recent years, the view that the utilities of particular health states are sufficiently consistent among individuals to provide an average value and a basis for rating health states has been gaining ground. In health economic analyses and EBM, utility is a measure of preference for a particular level or state of health; in other words, the benefits arising from being in the preferred state. Its measurement is difficult but one approach is to ask the individual what proportion of his normal life expectancy he would be willing to trade off to retain a particular health state (e.g. ability to see). The utilities we assign to particular health states are affected by our personal circumstances (e.g. age and occupation). For example, executives are willing to assign a higher utility to preserving normal speech than fire-fighters. Utilities are usually scaled to values in the range 0–1.

Perhaps the most widely known utility scale is the **Rosner and Watts matrix** in which a state of health characterized by an absence of disability and freedom from stress is given the maximum weight of 1. Being chairbound and in a state of severe stress is assigned a value of zero while being bed-ridden and in severe distress is given a negative score of –1.5.

Alternative methods for eliciting utilities include: (i) use of an analogue rating scale (0 = death, 1 = perfect health and values in between represent varying degrees of ill health); (ii) time trade-off whereby patients are asked to say how many years of their remaining lives they would be willing to forgo to regain complete health; (iii) standard gamble whereby patients are asked to choose between living the rest of their lives in their current state or a gamble which, if won, will mean perfect health and, if lost, will mean death. The probability of winning the gamble is altered until the point of indifference is reached.

Utility theory

Utility theory or expected utility theory is a formal model, first proposed by **von Neumann** and Morgenstern to deal with choice in the presence of risk. They described a set of axioms (see below) for characterizing rational behaviour and proposed a strategy for choosing among alternatives under such circumstances.

When measuring utilities, the person's risk preference is assumed to follow the following five axioms:

- *Completeness.* When choosing between two outcomes (o_1, o_2) there are three possibilities: o_1 is preferred to o_2, neither is preferred or o_2 is preferred to o_1.

- *Transitivity.* If o_1 is preferred to o_2 and o_2 is preferred to o_3, then o_1 should be preferred to o_3. Likewise, if o_2 and o_1 are considered equivalent and o_3 and o_2 are considered similarly, then o_1 and o_3 should be equivalent too.

- *Continuity.* If o_1 is preferred to o_2 and o_2 to o_3, then there exists a probability p that the lottery shown in Figure 27 is preferred to the certainty of receiving outcome o_2.

- *Independence* (or substitution). If o_1 and o_2 are equally attractive under conditions of certainty, then the lottery shown in Figure 27 and the lottery shown in Figure 28 will be equally attractive for any value of p or o_3.

- *Reduction of compound lotteries.* A lottery whose initial outcomes are themselves lotteries (i.e. a compound lottery) is as attractive as the simple lottery that is obtained when multiplying through probabilities as shown in Figures 29 and 30.

From those axioms, the expected utility (EU) theorem follows: a utility function U can be defined on the outcomes with the property that a choice with a higher expected utility is always preferred to one with a lower expected utility (von Neumann J, Morgenstern O (1947) *Theory of games and economic behavior*. 2nd edn. John Wiley, New York).

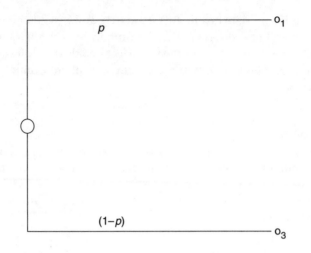

Figure 27 Lottery I

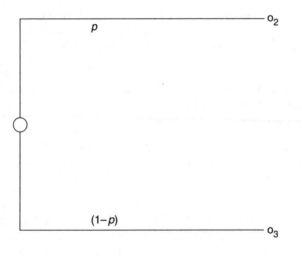

Figure 28 Lottery II

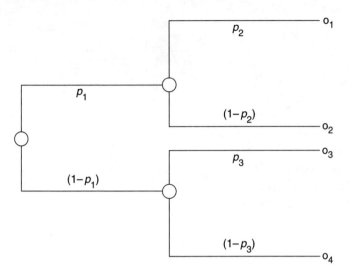

Figure 29 Lottery III

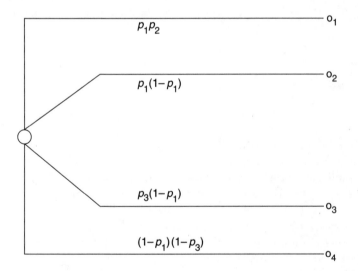

Figure 30 Lottery IV

Utilization management

Utilization management is a system for managing use of medical services, usually within a managed care organization, by a variety of techniques such as **pre-certification** and use of expert second opinion prior to sanctioning a request.

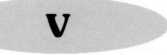

V

Variance

Variance is a measure of the spread of a distribution. If in a population of N individuals the measurements are x_i with i = 1 to N and the mean is μ then the variance σ^2 is given by:

$$\sigma^2 = \frac{\sum\limits_{i=1}^{N}(x_i - \bar{x})^2}{N}$$

In practice, population variances are estimated using samples of, say, size n. To reflect the reduced precision, the variance is then estimated by s^2:

$$s^2 = \frac{\sum\limits_{i=1}^{n}(x_i - \bar{x})^2}{n-1}$$

Variance inflation factor (VIF)

A measure of how much the variance associated with a coefficient of a statistical model is inflated by the lack of **orthogonality** (predictor variables correlated) in the design. The standard error of a model coefficient is increased by a factor equal to the square root of the VIF, when compared to the corresponding standard error in an orthogonal model. VIF values greater than 10 indicate that the coefficients are poorly estimated due to **multicolinearity** (presence of correlated predictor variables in the model). A coefficient with a VIF of 25 has a standard error which is five times higher than it would be if the design were orthogonal.

VIF (see **Variance inflation factor**)

von Neumann, John (1903–57)

John von Neumann was born in Hungary and moved to the United States in 1931 where he became a professor of mathematics and physics. He is credited with the development of game theory. His book, *The Theory of Games and Economic Behavior*, which he co-authored with Oskar Morgenstern (1902–77), is regarded as a classic in the subject. In addition to his major contributions to the development of economic theory, he also made important contributions in cybernetics and hence the development of the modern computer and atomic physics.

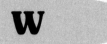

Welfare economics (*see under* **Positive economics**)

Willingness to pay

Willingness to pay is a technique for measuring how much people are prepared to pay for various outcomes so that these values can be incorporated into cost-benefit analyses (O'Brien B, Viramontes JL (1994) Willingness to pay: a valid and reliable measure of health state preference? *Medical Decision Making*. **14**: 289–97).

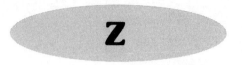

Z

Z variate

A random variable which is normally distributed with a mean of zero and a standard deviation of unity (also referred to as a variable with a standard normal distribution). It is common practice to convert other normally distributed variates to the standard normal so that the significance probability of sample observations from any normally distributed population can be obtained by reference to a single table of critical values (*see under* **Effect size**).